RUNNING TO YOU

AMELIA KRABACH

For Sean

CHAPTER ONE

L indsey Paulson knew her life could be better, but fear kept her stuck in a mundane routine. She wasn't in control of anything. Every Saturday morning, her father expected her at Jon's Diner for breakfast. Her mother assumed Lindsey was available to call back immediately, even when she was buried in work. And her friends? They expected her to drop everything for last-minute plans. Lindsey hated what her life had become. Her only solace was her best friend, Ida, who lived all the way in Phoenix, Arizona. Unfortunately, Lindsey was stuck in the Midwest, and their connection existed solely through their phones. They talked almost ten times a day.

"I hate my life!" Lindsey shouted into the phone as Ida's voicemail picked up yet again. "Where the heck are you?" She hung up and began pacing in front of her mirror. "I'm so fat," she muttered, glaring at her reflection. "Why can't anything ever go my way?" A sudden thought struck her. "Crap, I was supposed to call Mom an hour ago. She's going to be pissed." She hurriedly dialed her mom's number. Just as her mother picked up, Ida's name flashed on the screen. Torn, Lindsey decided to stick with her mom first.

"Hi, Mom, you called?"

"Yes, Lindsey, I did. What took you so long to call me back?" her mother asked, her tone curt. As her mom spoke, Lindsey's mind raced, trying to figure out how to end the conversation quickly so she could call Ida back. "So, what is it you need?" Lindsey asked impatiently. "Well, I need you to help can tomatoes at Aunt Mary's tomorrow. I told her we'd be there by 7 p.m. I'll pick you up at 6:30. See you then."

The last thing Lindsey wanted was to spend her evening canning tomatoes, but there was no arguing with her mom. Resigned, she mumbled an agreement and hung up.

She immediately called Ida. "Finally! Thank God I got a hold of you! I've been dying to talk to you all day!"

Ida laughed. "What's up?"

Lindsey let out a long sigh. "I hate my life, I'm so freaking fat, I wish I had a boyfriend, and the last thing I want to do tomorrow is can effing tomatoes."

Ida chuckled. "Oh, is that all?"

Lindsey smirked at the sarcasm but felt the frustration bubble up again. "Seriously, nothing is going right."

"Is anything going right in your life?" Ida teased, her tone lighthearted.

"Well, my job is okay, I guess. Except for the fact that I work too many hours."

Ida decided to shift the conversation. "Why don't you join a gym?" she suggested.

Lindsey groaned. "You know I can't do that. My jerk of an ex-boyfriend works at the one near my house, and the next closest one is a 35-minute drive. I'd be lucky to get there once a month."

Ida paused for a moment. "Well, there's an open road right outside your door. Why not go for a run?"

Lindsey stopped to think. Ida was right. Her neighborhood

was full of sidewalks, and with spring just beginning, it was the perfect time to be outdoors.

"What should I do? Just... start running?"

"Not exactly," Ida replied. "Why don't you start by walking for a bit, and then jog when you feel ready?"

Lindsey nodded, her mind warming to the idea. "Hmm... I think I might actually take your advice. I'll call you later—after my so-called 'run.'"

CHAPTER TWO

I t was a crazy idea—yes, a crazy idea. No wonder Lindsey hadn't even attempted the run after Ida suggested it the day before. But on her way home from work the next day, she began to reconsider. Her life was already full of crazy, from her unpredictable routines to the wireless phone job she loved. Why not add this to the list?

First, though, she needed her shoes. Surely, they were somewhere in her closet. She resolved to go for a run, to become one of those crazy runners she often saw outside. But as she rummaged through her things, she realized her running shoes were nowhere to be found. Frustrated but undeterred, she decided her old tennis shoes would have to do.

Throwing on a pair of sweats, an old t-shirt, and her worn-out shoes, Lindsey headed out the door for her first-ever run. Her plan was simple: start slow. She'd walk for ten minutes to build stamina, then jog for 30 seconds. It seemed manageable enough.

As she walked through her neighborhood, she couldn't help but notice how nice everything looked that day. After what felt like ten minutes, she decided it was time. "Any minute now, I'll be a runner," she thought to herself. "Okay, two minutes from now, I'll be a runner. Alright, here I go…"

She began jogging down her block, counting to herself, "One Mississippi, two Mississippi, three Mississippi…" By the ten-second mark, she felt ready to quit. "Come on, girl, keep it together," she thought. "You can do this for 30 frickin' seconds!"

Despite the huffing and puffing, Lindsey managed to push through, completing her 30-second jog. For a first attempt, it wasn't bad. "Okay," she told herself, "I need a 10-minute cool down, and I'm done. Wow, I just ran for the first time!"

Excited, she immediately called Ida to share the news. "Hey, Ida, I did it!" she exclaimed.

"You ran? For how long?" Ida asked.

"About two minutes," Lindsey replied, stretching the truth. She couldn't bring herself to admit that she barely made it past 30 seconds. "Tomorrow," she thought to herself. "Tomorrow, I'll run for two minutes—if I can find my running shoes."

As Lindsey ended the call, her mom arrived to pick her up. Still in her running attire, she made a quick change. A shower wasn't necessary—she hadn't even broken a sweat. Moments later, she was in the car, heading to Aunt Mary's to can tomatoes.

Aunt Mary's house was the usual setting for family gather-ings, which often involved producing something in bulk—like canned tomatoes. The process felt more like factory work, with everyone assigned a specific task to repeat for hours. Lindsey never understood why her family found it fun. After all, store-bought canned tomatoes were readily available, and the evening could have been spent relaxing instead.

Still, she didn't have the heart to tell her mom no, so there she was, peeling the skins off boiling tomatoes—a task she'd be doing for the next few hours. The bright spot of the evening was spending time with Aunt Joann. Joann, with her cheerful and encouraging personality, always managed to make everyone feel good, even when they didn't know they needed it.

As the night progressed, Lindsey mentioned her running attempt to Joann. Their conversation eventually turned to the upcoming spring carnival in town.

"You know, Lindsey," Joann said, "there's a race at the spring carnival called the Spring Chicken. I ran it 20 years ago. You should run it too!"

Lindsey vaguely remembered Joann running that race, and how her family had gathered to cheer her on during the parade. Before she knew it, the words had escaped her mouth: she would sign up for the race. It was as if time slowed down, and she could only watch as her family began congratulating her on her "achievement." Somehow, in the course of peeling tomatoes, she had committed to running a race—and now her family planned to be there to watch.

On the ride home with her mother, Lindsey reflected on the night. She had six jars of canned tomatoes, a race to train for, and a growing sense of anxiety. To top it off, she realized she'd probably spend the rest of the night on Amazon, buying running books, shoes, and gear—none of which she even knew how to pick.

CHAPTER THREE

John Stokely's newly purchased house was in a community that seemed perfect by his standards. Recently promoted in his engineering job and transferred to this area, he appreciated how close the house was to his workplace. Even better, it was within walking distance of bars and restaurants and surrounded by wooded areas ideal for his favorite pastime: mountain biking.

One of his favorite features was the large front window in his bungalow, which let in plenty of natural light and offered a great view of the entire neighborhood. At first, he thought it was strange to have the kitchen at the front of the house, but as he stood there putting away dishes, he realized the previous owners were onto something. It was smart, he thought. Instead of staring at a blank wall while spending so much time in the kitchen, he could look out at the lively street.

The house also boasted a wraparound porch, giving him a sense of privacy without blocking the big window. Elegant burning bushes lined the porch, adding a touch of charm. He was especially thankful that the house—and the landscaping— was in move-in-ready condition.

As he was finishing up in the kitchen, John noticed something odd across the street: his neighbor was lying on the ground in her yard. Without hesitation, he slipped on his shoes and hurried over to see what was wrong. She explained that she had been carrying groceries to her car when she slipped on one of her kids' tennis balls. Groceries were scattered across the yard.

As John helped gather the spilled items, a woman approached, clearly out of breath.

"Do you need help? Is anyone hurt?" the newcomer, Lindsey, asked between gasps.

The neighbor quickly assured both of them that she was fine, save for a bruised ego. The three of them laughed as they picked up the rest of the bruised fruit and scattered groceries.

John couldn't help but notice how intriguing this random stranger was. Lindsey, after introducing herself, resumed her jog down the street, wondering about the helpful man. How lucky, she thought, was that woman to have such a kind husband? Why couldn't she meet someone like that?

After helping his neighbor carry the groceries inside, John returned to his own house to finish tidying up the kitchen.

Lindsey, meanwhile, was attempting her second run. She was equipped with a new pair of running shoes and a book titled *Running in the Flow*, which encouraged runners to experience their runs by finding a state of flow. But there was no flow, not for Lindsey. She kept stopping to catch her breath, struggling to focus on her knees, shoulders, or feet as the book suggested. It all felt impossible.

Her mind kept wandering back to the gorgeous man helping his wife in the yard. Well, at least thinking about him made the run go by faster. Before she knew it, she was already back home.

Her second run wasn't as bad as she feared. Sure, she was sweaty and out of breath, but she was still alive. And that, for now, was enough.

CHAPTER FOUR

It was dark—pitch black—and the only thing illuminated were the bright pink running shoes pounding the pavement. Two weeks into running, and she was still going at a snail's pace. Part of the struggle was waking up at this ungodly hour, and the other part was learning how to run without injuring herself. At least her shins had finally stopped hurting, thanks to the basic advice she picked up from *Running in the Flow*, chapter two: tie your shoes correctly.

Why, she wondered, had she agreed to sign up for the Spring Chicken race? Yet here she was, dragging herself through sleep-deprived mornings with another month left to train. On the bright side, her runs gave her a new perspective on her neighborhood. Her apartment sat snugly among a mix of redeveloped homes, part of an area becoming trendy again. Normally, she sped through these streets in her car, heading to work, grabbing coffee, or meeting friends at a bar or restaurant. But now, running gave her time to notice the details: the corner house on this street had new furniture, and halfway up the other side of the block was the house where the hot guy lived—the one she had seen helping his wife that day.

The street was quiet this morning, with hardly any lights on. Good thing, too, because she was about to collapse onto the curb. "Just need a moment to check my schedule," she told herself, granting permission to take a break. Exhaustion weighed on her. One mile down, and this spot seemed like a good turnaround point—again. She sat on the curb, pulling out her phone. First, she scrolled through emails, then peeked at her schedule, and eventually played one, maybe two, games of Hearts. Time slipped away. She was in her own little world, proud for even getting out of bed but dreading the walk—or run—back. When she finally stood up, she realized she'd wasted a full half hour. Now she risked being late for work.

Running under a time limit wasn't fun, she mused, especially since races were all about time and finishing—two things she couldn't stand. Ironically, those were also the exact reasons she had signed up for the race. "Ha," she thought bitterly. "I hate them both."

Fortunately, work was a bright spot in her day. Unlike most people, she genuinely enjoyed her job and her coworkers, who made the workplace feel lighthearted and fun. Today was no exception.

Arriving late to the staff meeting, she was immediately "volunteered" for coffee duty. Jokes about the latecomer being punished flew around the room, all in good humor. Of course, the real joke was on them—she added sugar to everyone's coffee, whether they wanted it or not. "Aren't I sweet?" she thought with a grin.

The meeting wrapped up just before lunch, leaving her some time to order food and catch up on personal errands. At the top of her list was officially signing up for the Spring Chicken race. Surprisingly, she was starting to look forward to it. She had worked up to running two miles already, and the race was only 3.1 miles—or so she thought. Her aunt Joann had run it, and now it was her turn.

But then she clicked on the event's festival page and froze.

The Spring Chicken wasn't a 5K. It was a 10K.

Six-point-two miles. Double what she had thought. How had she been so wrong? Her aunt had made it sound like a short, easy race! Six-point-two miles wasn't short—it was practically a marathon in her mind.

"Have I bitten off more than I can chew?" she whispered to herself, staring at the screen.

She hurriedly dialed her aunt, and to her surprise, the call was answered on the first ring. The entire conversation felt like a blur. Her aunt casually confirmed that, yes, she had run the full 6.2 miles—laughing as she added that it was nothing compared to a marathon's grueling 26.2 miles.

Her stomach dropped.

Not only had she told her family she was running the Spring Chicken race, but now she was officially committed to running 6.2 miles.

Six. Point. Two.

She stared at the wall, her thoughts spiraling.

This is crazy.

I'm crazy.

What have I done?

It had barely been two weeks since she'd started running. Two weeks, and now she was signed up for a race double the distance she thought she could handle.

Lindsey grabbed her laptop and started frantically Googling beginner 10K training plans. Words like *intervals, tempo runs,* and *cross-training* flashed across her screen. It all sounded intimidating and a bit overwhelming. She finally settled on a plan that promised to get her to the finish line without dying, which, at this point, was all she could hope for.

"Okay, Lindsey," she muttered to herself, "one day at a time. You've got this... probably."

The next morning, she woke before sunrise, laced up her

shoes, and headed out the door. The air was crisp and the streets were quiet, except for the faint rustle of leaves

CHAPTER FIVE

Lindsey had downloaded a 10K training schedule from a website. Whether or not it was legitimate, she couldn't be sure. When starting from scratch, even the smallest crumb of advice from the internet felt like absolute truth.

This particular Saturday called for a long run—four miles, to be exact. Lindsey had cleverly planned her route to the halfway point at Jon's Diner, where she would meet her parents for breakfast. A free meal at the finish line? She couldn't pass that up.

Another early weekend morning meant no sleeping in, but she was determined. Her parents expected her at 8 a.m., and she still hadn't quite mastered pacing herself. To make things more bearable, she decided to spice it up with music. Scrolling through her playlist, she set it to shuffle, hoping for something upbeat. Instead, *September* by Earth, Wind & Fire began to play.

Not exactly the club music she had in mind, but the snappy rhythm quickly lifted her spirits. Before long, Lindsey was clapping along to the beat, adding a little flair to her run. She experimented with clapping clockwise, then to the left, then to the right, and soon she had choreographed a full routine in her head. The song was so catchy that she hit repeat, letting it play again and again as her feet hit the pavement.

A few blocks away, John was pedaling down the street on his way to the wooded trails for a morning bike ride. The sunrise painted everything in warm hues, and he felt content. That was until he noticed the runner ahead—a woman clapping and jogging, her energy infectious. It made him chuckle. Why couldn't he be as carefree as that?

As he drew closer, biking parallel to her from across the street, he realized it was the same woman who had helped his neighbor gather her groceries. He also remembered spotting her sitting on the curb in front of his house earlier in the week. Who was she? She seemed interesting, yet he couldn't summon the nerve to wave or cross the street. Instead, he kept riding, watching as she disappeared into Jon's Diner.

Inside the diner, Lindsey joined her parents just in time to catch them sipping their second cup of coffee. The breakfast was hearty, and her parents couldn't stop praising her for running all the way there. Lindsey felt proud, too. It was that same sense of pride that led her to agree—without much thought—to join the family on Sunday for their usual tamale-making assembly line.

Sunday would be another day spent cleaning corn husks for hours in her family's self-proclaimed "factory." Why did she always say yes to this sort of thing? It was a question she pondered on her run home.

The return trip was rough—running on a full stomach turned out to be a terrible idea. Lindsey alternated between jogging and walking, using the time to reflect on her tendency to agree to things without considering the consequences. Still, she managed to make it back, slightly queasy but with her dignity intact.

As she collapsed onto her couch, she realized one thing: she was committed now. Family tamales or not, the 10K was coming, and she'd better be ready.

CHAPTER SIX

By the time Lindsey hit the halfway point of her training plan, the realization of what she had committed to began to sink in. The four-mile run to Jon's Diner had been her longest distance yet, and it felt monumental—both physically and mentally. Yet, as she stared at the rest of the schedule on her fridge later that evening, she couldn't ignore the daunting increase in mileage looming ahead. The halfway point meant progress, but it also meant the real challenge was just beginning.

Her legs were beginning to adjust to the constant pounding, and the shin splints that plagued her early runs were finally fading. She wasn't fast, not by any stretch, but she was steady. Each run had become a mix of self-doubt and surprising break-throughs. Some mornings she woke up convinced she couldn't do it, only to find herself halfway through a run, feeling stronger than ever.

This newfound strength gave her a sense of pride, even if she still laughed at herself for overcommitting. The Spring Chicken Race wasn't just a test of endurance; it was a test of her willpower and her ability to follow through on something that once seemed impossible.

On the next Saturday morning, Lindsey decided to map out a new route, one that included a long loop through the park. It was a path she'd always driven past but had never taken the time to explore. Now, as her sneakers crunched on the gravel trail, she felt a small thrill at experiencing something new. The air smelled of damp earth and freshly cut grass, and the occasional cyclist or dog walker waved as she passed.

The halfway point of her run that day was marked by a bench overlooking a small pond. She stopped briefly, leaning forward with her hands on her knees as she caught her breath. The reflection of the morning sun on the water was peaceful, and for the first time in weeks, she allowed herself to pause and appreciate how far she'd come.

It wasn't perfect—her legs were sore, and she still struggled to keep her pace consistent—but she was doing it. Step by step, mile by mile, she was proving to herself that she could tackle this race.

As she headed home, Lindsey found herself wondering about that guy she kept seeing—the one from the yard full of groceries strewn everywhere and the mountain bike. She couldn't shake the feeling that their paths would cross again. But for now, her focus was on the road ahead—both in running and in life.

The halfway point wasn't just a marker on a schedule; it was a turning point in her mindset. She wasn't just running anymore—she was training. And somehow, that made all the difference.

CHAPTER SEVEN

The evening before the Spring Chicken 10K race, Lindsey was buzzing with a mix of nerves and excitement. She had spent the week obsessing over the details—her new running shoes, her carefully crafted playlist, and even the timing of her pre-race meal. But as the clock ticked closer to the evening, she found herself standing in front of her closet, pulling on a pair of jeans instead of her running gear.

It had been a long week at work, and her coworkers were eager to unwind. The group had been planning to go to TJ's, a local bar known for its excellent dirty martinis, and Lindsey had been invited. She'd hesitated at first, worried that one drink would set her off track for the race tomorrow, but the thought of spending the night with her friends was too tempting.

"My coworkers invited me out tonight at TJ's, and I'm thinking I might just go over for one," she said confidently over the phone to Ida.

"One?" Ida replied incredulously. "Isn't TJ's the place with the best dirty martinis? And that happens to be your favorite drink? Come on, I hardly think you'll stop at one!"

Lindsey laughed, feeling her resolve weaken. "I know, I know. But I've got the race tomorrow. I want to be fresh. This is my first 10K, and I can't show up hungover."

"Really?" Ida said, the sarcasm dripping from her voice. "You're going out with your sales team—who you have so much fun with—and you're really going to have just one martini? That's funnier than you running!"

Lindsey hesitated. "Okay, maybe I'll have *two*," she admitted. "But I'll stop there. I can't be sluggish tomorrow."

Ida wasn't convinced. "Alright, call me after the race and let me know how 'one martini' goes," she said, still skeptical.

After hanging up, Lindsey convinced herself that she could stick to her plan. She could just have a couple of drinks, chat with her friends, and head home early enough to get a good night's sleep. No big deal.

When she arrived at TJ's, the lively buzz of the bar hit her immediately. A few coworkers were already outside, puffing on cigars as they chatted and laughed. *Oh no*, she thought. *They're already on cigars and it's only 6 p.m. This could be a long night.*

But Lindsey pushed that thought aside and walked in, ordering her first dirty martini. As she joined her coworkers at a set of bar tops in the martini room, everything felt fun and carefree. She was starting to unwind, enjoying the conversations, the laughter, and the buzz of the bar. *Just one more drink,* she thought, *and then I'll leave.*

But as the night wore on, she excused herself to use the restroom. When she came back, there was a fresh martini waiting for her at her seat.

"Who ordered this?" she asked, glancing around at her coworkers. No one responded.

"Okay, okay," Lindsey said with a sigh, *one more,* she thought. "This will be the last one. I promise."

But by the time she reached her third martini, she realized she was in trouble. The warm, familiar feeling of the drinks and the laughter around her had taken over, and she'd completely lost track of her original plan. She was now on her fourth martini.

"Oh, no," she muttered to herself. She checked her phone— *10:30 p.m.* She had no way of getting home. She couldn't drive, so she ordered an Uber, hoping the ride would be quick. But somehow, while waiting for the ride, she managed to drink yet another martini. *Four*—Ida had been right. She couldn't believe it.

Sighing, Lindsey slumped into the back of the Uber. "I am so screwed," she muttered. How was she going to run tomorrow? She closed her eyes, bracing herself for the long, painful morning ahead.

CHAPTER EIGHT

Beep, beep, beep. That's the only sound echoing in Lindsey's head at this moment. She's dreaming that she's driving in New York, and all the cars are honking at her because she can't get her car out of first gear. She's driving a stick shift in the chaos of the city, and it's all a disaster.

Suddenly, Lindsey stirs and slowly starts to realize she's not in the car—she's in her bed. The beeping is just her alarm, and oh no, she forgot to plug it in last night. Who knows how much battery she has left? And worse, it's race day. *Oh crap, it's race day.*

Her head is pounding, her mouth is dry, and it feels like the universe is conspiring against her. It's only 5:40 a.m., though, and she has a few hours to pull this off before the 9:00 a.m. race.

She gets up, splashes some cold water on her face, throws her hair into a messy bun, and gulps down a huge glass of water. Her head spins, but she pushes through. Then, reality hits again —her car is still parked at the bar from last night. Great. Another kink in her already chaotic morning.

Lindsey starts the coffee maker. If nothing else, that might help clear her foggy brain. Who's even up this early? *Who can I call to help me?* Then it hits her: Aunt Joann is an early riser. Perfect. She takes the next hour to figure out what to wear for the race, all while nursing a 3-4 martini hangover—she's not even sure if she finished that fourth one.

At 6:30, Aunt Joann shows up, beaming, as usual. Lindsey loves how unjudgmental Joann is. She climbs into the car, and they head to the bar to retrieve her vehicle. After that, Joann kindly drops Lindsey off in the isolated parking lot of one vehicle and tells her she will see her at the race later.

Lindsey heads to the race venue, where packet pickup is running from 7 a.m. to 9 a.m. She arrives early, knowing it's her first race and she's a little lost. At the registration table, she gets her race bib, and it's time to pin it on. Simple, right? Not exactly. It takes her three attempts to get the safety pins in without the bib flapping awkwardly. *Next time, I'll pin this before putting on the shirt,* she tells herself, shaking her head.

With the bib on, she has about an hour to kill. She watches the other runners stretch, adjust their laces, and get their music ready. Lindsey does none of this. She's still feeling the remnants of last night's hangover, and she's not sure what she's doing. Her phone is on 23% battery, though, so she heads to the charging station to juice it up. *At least I'll have music for the run,* she thinks.

As the crowd grows, Lindsey weaves her way toward the starting line. She notices the row of porta-potties and, of course, she now has to go. She didn't need to earlier, but the sight of the long line now triggers the need. She starts pacing, feeling her stomach churn. It's a mix of race nerves and last night's nachos. But the line is so long. She's stressing about making it in time for the race, too.

She's starting to panic when the person in front of her turns around and starts talking. She's funny, making fun of herself and the whole running community. Her humor eases Lindsey's nerves, and she relaxes, realizing the pressure is all self-inflicted.

"Just have fun," the woman says before heading into the next stall.

Lindsey smiles to herself. *Just have fun,* she repeats in her head. She gets into the next stall, quickly releases all the anxiety that's been building up, and takes a deep breath. It's quick, and she's just in time. The race has started, and the crowd begins to move toward the starting line.

I'm actually doing this, Lindsey thinks as she heads to the start. All she needs to do is have fun.

CHAPTER NINE

Lindsey started off running faster than she should have. The excitement of the race was contagious, and she got swept up in the crowd, moving at a pace that felt too quick for her but seemed to be the rhythm of everyone around her. *This is way faster than I usually go,* she thought, but as the other runners continued, she felt compelled to keep up. After a while, though, her body told her to slow down. She eased into a more comfortable pace, and soon, she noticed something: the faces around her weren't all serious anymore. They were smiling. Maybe it was her imagination, or maybe running slower allowed her to become more present in the moment. Either way, it didn't matter. She had already passed the first mile marker, and that was something she hadn't expected. *Thank you, mind,* she thought. *Now just five more to go.*

Mile two felt a little more fun, and she found herself enjoying the supporters cheering along the way. Some held up signs, including one that said "Power Up Here!" with a circle in the middle to place a hand on for an energy boost. While she didn't feel a sudden surge of energy, the gesture was fun, and it got her to mile two. Maybe there was something to it after all.

By mile three, she saw her family. Her mom, her aunts, and her dad stood along the side, cheering her on with high fives and enthusiastic support. It gave her a burst of energy that carried her through to the halfway point. As she turned around to head back, her phone started ringing, and it was Ida calling on FaceTime. *Of course,* Lindsey thought, as she answered.

Ida, still in bed due to the three-hour time difference, was as funny as ever, pointing out little details like the sound of Lindsey's breathing, the runner behind her, and even making light of the supporters, who were now the family cheering her on for the second time. At times, Ida didn't even say anything; she just stayed on the phone, her presence calming Lindsey's nerves. That simple connection helped Lindsey power through the next mile. When they got to almost mile five, Lindsey thanked Ida and let her go, plugging her music back in to carry her through the final stretch.

The last mile felt like a challenge, but Lindsey was determined. She focused on staying present, trying to enjoy the moment and have fun. And then, as if on cue, the 6-mile sign appeared in front of her. *It's almost over,* she thought, feeling a surge of excitement. The sound of the finish line music and the announcer calling out the names of finishers fueled her adrenaline. She started to pick up her pace, but then, she realized something was wrong. *Where's my family?* She scanned the crowd and couldn't see them. *Where's the finish line?*

She began to panic. *This doesn't make sense,* she thought. *I'm almost there, why is this part the hardest?* The final .2 miles, the shortest part of the race, seemed to stretch on forever. Her chest tightened, and she fought the urge to walk, but her legs felt like lead.

And then, she saw it—the finish line. A rush of adrenaline surged through her, and she found herself running faster than she ever thought possible. She had no idea where the energy came from, but suddenly, her legs were moving at lightning speed. She could see her family cheering on the sidelines, and she waved to them as she pushed through the final stretch, crossing the finish line with a burst of joy.

"I did it," she whispered to herself, though she could barely feel her legs anymore. They felt like rubber beneath her, but it didn't matter. She had finished.

A volunteer placed the coveted medal with a large chicken on it around her neck, and Lindsey felt a wave of accomplishment. She was proud, but her body was quickly reminding her that it was time for a rest. She made her way through the vendor area, collecting free food, drinks, and race swag, though she could barely focus on any of it. The only thing on her mind now was the free massage.

Lindsey hobbled to the tent where the massage therapists were set up, and she sank into the chair with relief. The massage was heavenly, and she felt herself unwinding with each stroke. The tent was festive, sponsored by the Space Alien Marathon, and people were congratulating each other, sharing stories of their races. There was so much positivity in the air, and amidst it all, Lindsey found herself signing up for the marathon.

It was a blur, but somehow, in the joy of the moment, she decided to do it. The marathon, scheduled for the fall, was just for her. It was something she wanted to do, just for herself. She didn't know what had gotten into her, but she knew this was her next big challenge. And somehow, after everything she had just experienced, it felt like the right decision.

CHAPTER TEN

Sunday morning crept in slowly, bringing with it a deep ache in Lindsey's muscles and an overwhelming sense of what she'd committed herself to the day before. She felt like a cement brick—exhausted, sore from that final sprint to the Spring Chicken finish line, and mentally numb from the realization that she'd signed up for a marathon.

A marathon. Twenty-six point two miles. What had she been thinking?

She shuffled to the kitchen to make coffee, her legs protesting every step, and stared blankly at the counter. She had five months to prepare for something that felt impossible. The thought alone was enough to make her want to crawl back into bed, but she had to start somewhere. Today, that meant cracking open the stack of running books she'd optimistically purchased months ago and never touched. Somewhere in those pages, she hoped, were the secrets to transforming her from a novice runner into someone who could conquer 26.2 miles without collapsing.

Once the coffee was brewed and steaming in her favorite mug, she settled onto the couch and started thumbing through the books. They were full of advice: running form, nutrition, gear, recovery. It was overwhelming, but she zeroed in on the one thing she could control right now—her training schedule. She grabbed a notebook and sketched out the bones of a plan, focusing first on when she could run.

Four running days, three rest days. That felt manageable, at least on paper. She quickly decided Saturdays would be one of her rest days; there was no way she'd run on Saturday mornings after a Friday night out. She made that mistake once and wasn't eager to repeat it. Tuesdays, Thursdays, Fridays, and Sundays would be her running days, with her longest runs scheduled for Fridays. Starting the weekend with a big effort felt ambitious, but it also left her Saturday and Sunday afternoons free to recover.

With the schedule drafted, Lindsey sat back and eyed it skeptically. It looked good in her notebook, but her first 10k had proven that she was far from prepared. She hadn't known how to pace herself, hadn't worn the right socks, and had barely trained consistently. This marathon would demand a whole new level of commitment and planning. Could she really stick to this?

The thought of failure loomed in the back of her mind, but she pushed it aside. She'd figure it out. For now, she had two goals: rest her aching legs and find a way to display her medal from the Spring Chicken race. She wandered over to the wall near her entryway, medal in hand, and started imagining where it might go. It felt silly, celebrating a 10k finish when she had a marathon looming, but she reminded herself it was still an achievement. The medal represented her first step into this crazy world of running.

For now, she would bask in that small victory, let her body recover, and focus on the task ahead. Training officially began Tuesday.

CHAPTER ELEVEN

The first day of Lindsey's marathon training was one for the books. The rain poured down relentlessly, but she couldn't let that stop her. It was Tuesday, and according to her training plan, there was no skipping. Even quitters don't quit on their first day, she told herself as she stepped outside, squinting against the storm. The weather seemed almost comical as it threw her into a situation she had never imagined herself in—running through a downpour, shoes drenched, hair plastered to her face. It felt almost like a cruel joke, but one she was determined to laugh through.

As the rain soaked her to the bone, her playlist didn't help but add a touch of absurdity to the moment. "I Love a Rainy Night" blared through her earbuds, the upbeat rhythm somehow adding a touch of fun to the miserable weather. The lyrics seemed oddly fitting, reminding her that if she didn't take the rain too seriously, maybe it wouldn't be so bad. But as she slogged through mile after mile, her shoes felt heavier with each step, like they were filled with lead.

The rain was relentless, turning the streets into rivers, and just when she thought things couldn't get worse, disaster struck.

As she approached a puddle that had formed into a small pond on the sidewalk, she miscalculated the jump to avoid it. Her foot slipped, sending her crashing to the ground in a mudslide. Her left side hit the wet earth with a sickening squelch—her knee, hand, and shoe now coated in thick, brown mud.

Lindsey groaned, but she knew she had no choice but to keep going. She picked herself up, brushed herself off, and continued on her run, trying to laugh at the situation. *This is insane,* she thought, but she wasn't about to quit. By the time she made it back to her apartment, she was a muddy mess. She trudged up the stairs and paused at the door, debating whether she was even going to make it inside without getting more dirt everywhere. In the end, she decided to peel off her soaked clothes right at the threshold, making a mental note to have a stash of rag towels handy for future muddy runs.

A quick shower later, Lindsey combed out her wet hair and scrambled to get on her sales Zoom call. Her coworkers were understanding, of course. They knew her well enough to see through her disheveled appearance, and it wasn't like she needed to impress them. After the meeting wrapped up, the conversation turned to her first training run, which had clearly been a mess. She joked about how a treadmill would have been a lifesaver in the downpour.

Brad, one of her coworkers, mentioned that his mom was getting rid of her treadmill and offered to give it to Lindsey for free. Mark, another colleague, chimed in, offering to help transport it with his truck. Lindsey, relieved that the universe was giving her a little break, agreed to the plan. The following day was supposed to be clear and sunny, making it the perfect time to pick up the treadmill.

She couldn't help but smile, grateful for her friends at work. Unlike her family, who often made her feel obligated to help and attend events, her coworkers seemed to just want to help because they cared. There was no pressure, just genuine kindness. But it made her think—maybe she needed to find a way to navigate her family relationships more like she did with her friends. That thought felt daunting, though. The last thing she wanted was to add another complicated layer to her already strained connections with them. Thank goodness for Aunt Joann, who was a breath of fresh air. She was the one family member Lindsey knew she could count on, and she needed to figure out how to build more relationships like that within her family.

The next afternoon, Lindsey met Brad and Mark to pick up the treadmill. When they arrived at Brad's mom's house, they found the 1980s-era treadmill sitting in the garage. It was a basic model—no fancy buttons, just the simple "ON" switch. Lindsey didn't mind, though. It was free, and it was exactly what she needed. The treadmill went into the truck, and they made their way back to Lindsey's apartment.

Up the stairs it went, straight into the living room. The space wasn't ideal, but it was the only place that had an outlet and enough room. *I'll have to figure something out for this weekend,* Lindsey thought, planning a trip to Home Depot for an extension cord. Mark had to try it out, of course, and seeing him attempt to run in his work clothes, only to fall off the treadmill, had Lindsey laughing. They spent the next hour chatting about work, sharing stories, and having a couple of drinks. The moment felt lighthearted, and Lindsey found herself wishing for more of these spontaneous, carefree moments—especially with someone she could share them with.

But deep down, she knew she wasn't ready for a relationship. Her breakup with Todd still weighed on her, and she wasn't yet ready to dive back into the dating scene. Her decision to start running outside, rather than at the gym, had been motivated by avoiding Todd. She was still adjusting to the idea of being single, navigating her own space. *Maybe someday,* she thought, *I'll be ready for someone new. But not now. Right now, it's just me.*

As she glanced at the treadmill in her living room, she realized that this was just one more step toward taking control of her life. She was figuring out who she was outside of relationships and the pressure of family obligations. For now, the treadmill was a reminder that she was on the right path, even if it wasn't always easy.

CHAPTER TWELVE

The next morning, rain pelted against Lindsey's window, signaling another day of soggy weather. On just her second day of marathon training, she wasn't about to let the weather win, so she decided to give the newly acquired treadmill in her living room a shot.

Lindsey headed to her laundry area to grab her workout clothes, only to discover that her one clean set had never made it to the dryer. Her backup set was still sitting in the wash basin, caked in dried mud from her first run. Fantastic, she thought, standing there in defeat. But she wasn't about to let a lack of clean clothes stop her.

After a quick internal debate, she decided running in her nude-colored bra and a black thong would suffice—no one was around to see her, after all. "Why not?" she said aloud, shrugging as she laced up her dirty, hot pink running shoes.

As soon as she started the treadmill, she felt surprisingly liberated. No restrictive clothing, just her body in motion. She smiled to herself. *Maybe people are onto something with this minimal running thing,* she thought. By the end of the first mile, she was feeling great. Her earbuds were in, music was pumping, and the steady rhythm of her feet on the treadmill felt almost meditative.

That is, until she glanced at herself in the mirror above her faux mantel. She froze mid-stride, catching sight of the absurd image staring back at her: a woman in a ratty, flesh-toned bra, a black thong, white socks, and glaringly pink shoes. It was an outfit worthy of its own comedy sketch, and Lindsey couldn't help but burst out laughing. The ridiculousness of the scene made her nearly lose her footing.

By mile two, the novelty had worn off. She was bored out of her mind. The treadmill was no longer a liberating machine of fitness but a torturous hamster wheel. She tried switching up her music, even imagining herself outdoors, but the monotony was suffocating. Just as she was about to throw in the towel, her phone rang.

It was Ida, her early-rising best friend on the West Coast. Lindsey eagerly picked up, glad for the distraction. "Running?" Ida asked as soon as Lindsey answered. "Why do you sound like you're on a conveyor belt?"

"That's because I *am* on a conveyor belt of death," Lindsey groaned. The call made the remaining two miles bearable as Ida peppered Lindsey with jokes and stories, a lifeline in the monotony.

As the run ended, Lindsey hopped off the treadmill and headed straight for the shower, relieved the ordeal was over. But as she scrubbed her skin clean of sweat, she noticed an uncomfortable stinging between her thighs and along her backside. Looking down, she realized the friction from running in her makeshift outfit had left her with raw, angry rashes. Her "brilliant" idea was now literally biting her in the ass.

She dried off and slathered herself in lotion, wincing with every touch. Her running books had mentioned something about chafing creams—something she clearly needed to pick up ASAP.

Sitting on her couch in fresh clothes, her gaze landed on the treadmill. "Never again," she muttered. The mind-numbing monotony was bad enough, but the post-run pain sealed the deal. She needed to figure out how to get rid of it. The thought of Brad or Mark taking it off her hands made her chuckle. She could already hear the jokes they'd crack.

For now, the treadmill sat there, a monument to her short-lived experiment in indoor running. Tomorrow, rain or shine, she'd be back outside. Even if it meant getting drenched, it was still better than this.

CHAPTER THIRTEEN

The next day brought Lindsey's first long run: an ambitious eight miles that felt daunting even before she tied her shoes. She slipped on her backpack full of water, unsure how much she'd actually need but erring on the side of caution. Fridays were light for her at work, so she planned to squeeze in the run during the quiet morning hours, keeping her phone nearby just in case.

Greased up with ointment from the aftermath of her treadmill run, she started out with a mix of nerves and determination. The first mile passed with only a slight irritation from her lingering rash. By mile three, however, she realized she had overestimated her hydration needs. Her bladder was full, and it was all she could think about. No bathrooms in sight. She was on a residential route with nothing but driveways and lawns—definitely not ideal.

You can hold it, she told herself. *Just focus on the run.* But the urgency grew unbearable, and when she spotted a cluster of trees and bushes off the main street, she decided to risk it. Sliding behind the cover of greenery, she crouched low and hoped no passing cars would notice her absence.

The relief was heavenly. The duration, however, felt like an eternity. *Why does it take forever when you're trying to be quick?* she thought as she scanned the area nervously. Finally, the ordeal ended, and she pulled up her pants, instantly reminded of her rash as the fabric scraped against her skin. She muttered under her breath, adjusted her waistband, and got back on the path.

By the turnaround point at mile four, her bladder was no longer an issue, but the irritation from her rash was intensifying. She tried tucking her shirt into her pants for cushioning, but the makeshift solution only lasted a minute before her shirt worked its way free. Next, she attempted widening her stance, hoping to reduce friction. It helped minimally, but the discomfort remained a nagging presence.

To distract herself, Lindsey cranked up her music and focused on the landmarks passing by. She hit mile six, marking the farthest she'd ever run in her life. Despite the discomfort and the earlier mishap, she felt a swell of pride. Just a few months ago, running even a single block had seemed impossible.

Slowing her water intake had worked, too. Her bladder was cooperating, and she felt a small sense of victory over that minor mistake. The rash, however, was still the boss of her day, making its presence known with every step. But with only a mile to go, Lindsey was determined to finish strong.

As she entered her neighborhood, the familiar streets gave her a mental boost. The moment she crossed the eight-mile mark—right at her apartment steps—relief and triumph washed over her. She had done it: her first long run. Exhausted, sore, and a little raw, she climbed the stairs, each step feeling like a monumental effort.

Now she had the rest of her day ahead—finishing reports, catching up on work, and bracing herself for the evening's plans. She and her coworkers were set to meet at a sports bar that happened to be her ex's usual haunt. It wasn't her choice, but the group rotated locations, and it was her turn to endure the awkwardness. Her plan: leave before 8 p.m., the time Todd typically rolled in, freshly showered and ready to socialize.

As she leaned against her apartment door, panting and sweaty, Lindsey smiled to herself. The run had been tough, but she'd survived—and now, nothing, not even the prospect of a Friday night run-in, could take away her sense of accomplishment.

CHAPTER FOURTEEN

The morning had started rough, thanks to the unexpected encounter with her ex the night before. Lindsey had timed her exit from the sports bar perfectly—or so she thought—but Todd had shown up earlier than expected. The awkwardness was palpable, despite her friends' best efforts to smooth things over. Seeing him again brought back memories of their five-year relationship, one that had dragged on too long. He'd always wanted her to change, to mold herself into his ideal partner, without doing any self-improvement of his own. She had loved him, but his lack of substance and refusal to grow had become unbearable. Her family had adored him, which made things worse. As much as she knew the breakup was for the best, it still stung.

This morning's breakfast with her dad was a small reprieve from her swirling emotions. Though she'd wanted to stay in bed, Lindsey forced herself up, threw on some clothes, and drove to the diner. Running to breakfast—something she'd once done as part of a training experiment—was decidedly off the table.

Her dad was in high spirits, likely because her mom was off

at a craft show with one of her sisters, Theresa. They had the morning mostly to themselves, aside from some friendly nods from his coffee buddies. Over pancakes and eggs, he filled her in on the latest family plans: a beet-pickling session her mom had penciled her into. Lindsey bit back a groan but nodded along. They briefly touched on her marathon training, and he expressed genuine surprise and admiration for her dedication. The conversation lightened her mood a little, though she avoided bringing up her ex—her dad had liked him far too much.

On her way home, Lindsey decided to call Aunt Joann to confirm the beet-pickling plans. Joann, her mom's youngest sister and an eternal source of wisdom and style, was enjoying a leisurely morning. She invited Lindsey to meet her at the local farmer's market, and Lindsey, already out and about, decided to join her.

The market was a hub of activity, a mix of trendy stalls and mid-century modern antiques. Lindsey quickly realized she was underdressed. Joann, ever polished even in casual clothes, greeted her with a smile and her neatly folded reusable bags. Lindsey admired her aunt—successful, independent, and effort-lessly chic. Joann had spent her career in finance, retired early, and now split her time between traveling and family gatherings. Lindsey often thought of her as the cool aunt, the one who somehow always knew the right thing to say or do.

The two meandered through the market, sampling coffee and admiring heirloom tomatoes. It was a relaxed, pleasant morning—until Lindsey spotted *him*. Across the way, a man she recognized was browsing jars of local honey. He was handsome in that effortless way, and worse, he caught Joann's attention too. She nudged Lindsey and pointed him out, commenting that he wasn't wearing a wedding ring. Lindsey's face flushed crimson as she quickly steered them to the next stall.

Joann gave her a questioning look. Lindsey sighed. "Yeah, I

noticed him, but he's married. A while back, I helped his wife when she fell with her groceries. Trust me, he's off-limits."

Joann raised her eyebrows, shrugged, and changed the subject. But the damage was done. As they shopped, Lindsey couldn't help but think about the man. It wasn't that she was interested—he was married, end of story—but there was something about the encounter that left her unsettled.

For the rest of the morning, Lindsey tried to shake the thought of him, focusing instead on her time with Joann and the haul of fresh produce they were gathering. Still, she couldn't help but think it was a shame he wasn't available. Maybe it was just the post-breakup sensitivity talking, but it felt like a cruel twist of fate. She brushed it off, determined not to dwell on something that wasn't hers to consider.

By the time they wrapped up their shopping and parted ways, Lindsey felt a little lighter. Her rough morning had smoothed into something calmer, and she was ready to face the rest of her weekend—even if it included pickling beets.

CHAPTER FIFTEEN

The second week of training was the same as the first week: short runs on Sunday, Tuesday, and Thursday, with a long run on Friday. It was the same amount of running—three miles and then eight miles on Friday. Lindsey remembered not to drink as much water on the long run this week, and she kept the same running routes to simplify things, especially since work was launching a new phone promotion and her days were going to be busy.

Each day before her run, she saluted her new running totem: *The TREADMILL.* Still sitting smack dab in the living room with no takers, it was super motivational to see the treadmill stare back at her as she left the house, rain or shine. It was a reminder that things could be much worse—she could be forced to run indoors. She'd also added a few more running shirts and pants to her wardrobe, ensuring she'd never face the "no clean clothes" debacle again. It felt like progress—small steps toward feeling like an actual runner.

That week, she also scheduled her trip to see Ida in Phoenix. It was Ida's 30th birthday in less than a month, and Lindsey knew she had to be there. Ida's fiancé was throwing an amazing surprise birthday party, and the only thing Ida knew was that Lindsey was coming to visit. Lindsey hoped it would stay a secret because Ida figured out *everything*. It was her superpower —nothing ever got past her.

Ida was enthusiastically planning what they would do while Lindsey was in town, and Lindsey had to go along with the planning, knowing full well that there was an entirely different plan in motion. She was glad her running schedule was staying consistent that week since the phone calls to Ida were becoming more and more precarious.

The phone promotion was also a *cluster fuck*. Phones had been shipped to the wrong locations, and some of the point-of-sale signage was backlogged. Lindsey was fielding angry calls from her distributors but feeling far less stressed than her usual crazed energy when these things happened. She realized her running was really helping with her stress levels. What normally would have been a "need to go to the bar and drink" kind of week was instead a week she took in stride, putting out as many fires as she could without being pushed to the brink. She was noticing a change—and in a good way.

CHAPTER SIXTEEN

I t was the Friday of Memorial Day weekend, and John Stokely still hadn't planted his two flats of flowers from the farmers market a few weeks back. Some of the flowers were starting to look pretty dilapidated. His new homeownership still lacked the necessary tools for planting. He really just needed to break down and buy the shovels and weeding tools required to finish the task.

His engineering background sometimes made it impossible to just go ahead and do something that wasn't researched and planned. This was why the flats still sat on the front porch. He needed to get out of his head and plant away. *This isn't a design,* he told himself.

If only he could be more like that blonde woman who ran by the house without a care in the world. He remembered seeing her at the farmers market. He thought he saw him as well, but she immediately turned around and went the other way. *It's probably because I'm too boring,* he thought to himself.

The only thing he did that wasn't boring was mountain biking. He was introduced to it a few years ago by a buddy and was instantly hooked. He loved adventure but needed a push to try new things. He was more reserved growing up with his big family of five and didn't really need to try much since most of his family did everything for him. That was the advantage of being the youngest with a big age difference. He was the "oops baby," and with the eight-year gap, it felt more like having a bunch of parents around.

When he moved to the Midwest, it was like he was an only child—and an adult—for the first time, since the rest of his family lived on the East Coast. It was a great decision because he was finally starting to come into his own. He was trying new things for the first time and learning homeownership without the intrusion of his older siblings. *This is a good thing,* he thought.

Though some days, like today, he wished his older sisters were around to tell him how to plant his flowers—or maybe even take over and plant them for him. Today, he told himself, he was going to head to the hardware store after work, get yard tools, and buy a spray nozzle for the hose left behind with the house to water the flowers.

Lindsey was on her long run that day. She had gotten up extra early that Friday since it was the long weekend. She had a bunch of work that needed to be done before the typical 3 p.m. rush to beat the long weekend traffic.

She wished she were heading out of town this weekend but was excited to at least be going to Phoenix the following weekend for Ida's birthday.

Today's run consisted of 10 miles. This was another first for her, but she considered last week's 9-mile run similar preparation. The only difference was the flavor of her electrolyte drink. This time, it was fruit punch. The grocery store was all out of cherry and berry blast, so fruit punch had to do.

She was using the information from her *Flow Running* book

and taking the time to "body sense." This helped immensely to slow down her pace and connect with herself. She first checked in with her feet, then her knees, then her hips, back, shoulders, and finally her mindset.

Sometimes she received hilarious feedback from herself—especially when she checked in on her mindset. There were generally a few curse words coming from that space, but overall, her body was accepting the miles and the run in general.

This Friday in particular, Lindsey had a companion in the form of Mr. Hiccup. Mr. Hiccup joined her at mile 4 and continuously annoyed her for the rest of the run. Lindsey tried jumping up and down, pulling on her ears, and taking deep breaths, but nothing worked. Mr. Hiccup proved to be a tried-and-true companion all the way to the end.

She also experienced left knee pain around the 8-mile marker, but it disappeared by mile 9. She was thankful because one annoying companion was enough.

She spent the last mile running through her favorite part of the neighborhood and tried to ignore Mr. Hiccup by checking out the current house updates on that street. One house, in particular, caught her eye: flats of flowers were still sitting on the porch, looking pretty pathetic.

If I had garden tools, she thought, *I'd have already planted them.*

Her run finished, and finally, Mr. Hiccup went on his way. She realized the fruit punch flavor was the culprit and decided to give away the rest of that six-pack to her coworkers.

CHAPTER SEVENTEEN

Today was finally the day she got to see her best friend, Lindsey thought to herself. It had been a short week since Monday was a holiday, and she had taken today off. All that stood between her and her flight to see Ida was her long run of 12 miles.

The run was already shaping up to be a challenge. She was overthinking—too many thoughts about what she had packed or forgotten to pack, how much she wished the run was already over, and, to top it off, a call during mile 6 about a work crisis. Her coworker didn't want to bother her but needed her expertise to handle the situation. Now, her mind was consumed with work, problem-solving, and packing worries.

By mile 8, the phantom knee pain in her left leg returned. She slowed to a walk and wanted to quit. She was still four miles from home, her knee was aching, her mind was stuck at work, and her soul was already on the plane to Phoenix.

It was awful. How could she focus? She stopped for a moment, looked around, and took in her surroundings. She gave herself a firm pep talk.

"Buckle up," she said aloud. "You can do this."

Somehow, something clicked. She started running again.

The knee pain disappeared, and she powered through her last three miles with renewed focus. She finished the run, climbed the stairs to her apartment, and saluted her treadmill as she passed it.

"See?" she reminded herself. "It's so much better to run outdoors."

Her treadmill had become more of a packing station. Hanging neatly from it were items she planned to pack into her suitcase, and now, her running shoes joined them at the base. All she had left to do was shower, get dressed, pack, and call an Uber to the airport.

LINDSEY ARRIVED AT THE AIRPORT EARLY, WHICH GAVE HER TIME to grab something to eat. She pulled out her phone to check in with Ida.

Ida, already deep into planning her birthday weekend, asked Lindsey to step up her game. Ida loved Lindsey's spontaneity since she herself was such a planner. She wanted Lindsey to come up with something special to kick off her 30th birthday celebration when she got off the plane.

Internally panicking, Lindsey agreed. She promised to come up with something, but now her supposedly relaxing flight to Phoenix felt like it would be spent brainstorming instead.

Surprisingly, the flight turned out to be inspirational. Lindsey's creativity started flowing, and she even cracked herself up. She came up with a plan: *30 things to do before you turn 30.* She started jotting down ideas for Ida to try—things she had never done before.

Since Ida was such a meticulous planner, Lindsey knew it would be hilariously fun to see her tackle a bunch of random activities. Their friendship had always thrived on Lindsey's playful energy and Ida's willingness to embrace the chaos.

As the plane neared Phoenix, Lindsey had to tone down her excitement to conserve energy for the wild night she had planned. She smiled, feeling proud of her plan and ready to celebrate Ida's big milestone.

CHAPTER EIGHTEEN

I da was already texting Lindsey before she even made it to baggage claim. Her messages were filled with funny memes about their weekend together and excitement about the surprise gift Lindsey had promised.

Ida wasn't easy to shop for—she was the kind of woman who had everything. Lindsey had chipped in with Ida's other friends to buy her an expensive pair of high heels she'd been eyeing, but Lindsey knew Ida expected something unique from her. That's how the idea of *30 Things to Do Before You Turn 30* was born.

When Lindsey slid into the passenger seat of Ida's car, Ida announced their first stop: margaritas at a nearby Mexican restaurant. "Then," she added, "you can tell me all about this gift of yours."

Lindsey had only managed to come up with 14 items for the list so far, but she figured a margarita might spark her creativity. She explained the idea to Ida, who burst out laughing and declared, "I'm all in!"

Lindsey asked if Ida's fiancé, Jeff, would be joining them. "Not yet," Ida replied. "He'll meet us back at the house later tonight. For now, it's just us."

The first item on the list was arm wrestling a stranger. Ida eagerly agreed, and soon, two older gentlemen sitting nearby—fresh from a round of golf—were roped into their fun. When they learned about the list, one of the men suggested grocery cart racing, which Ida confessed she'd never done before.

Minutes later, the group was at a nearby market, laughing uproariously as the two older men pushed Lindsey and Ida in grocery carts through the parking lot.

Their night continued at a bowling alley, where one of the gentlemen happened to know the owner. Inside, the antics escalated. Ida poured drinks behind the bar, sang with the live band, splashed water in Lindsey's face, and checked off a string of other firsts from the list.

The night was a blast, but as it got late, Lindsey reminded Ida they should head home—Jeff would be waiting for them and had no idea what they'd been up to.

As they were leaving the bowling alley, they spotted something that stopped them in their tracks: a gleaming red Lamborghini pulling out of the parking lot. Ida admitted she had never driven or even sat in a Lamborghini before, so Lindsey convinced her to ask the owner if she could take it for a spin.

To their surprise, the owner, amused by their quest, agreed—on the condition that he rode along. Ida hopped into the driver's seat while Lindsey stayed back, snapping pictures as they cruised around the lot.

Moments later, Ida turned a corner and disappeared out onto the street. When she finally returned a few minutes later, she screeched to a stop in front of Lindsey, grinning ear to ear. It seemed like the perfect end to her night—or so they thought.

Out of nowhere, five police cars and an unmarked vehicle swarmed the lot, surrounding the Lamborghini. Lindsey and Ida watched in disbelief as the situation unfolded.

The car, it turned out, had no license plates and was brand

new. Police assumed it had been stolen, and when Ida took it out onto the street, it looked like she was fleeing the scene in a stolen vehicle.

Two hours later, after sitting on the curb and answering questions, the mix-up was finally cleared up. Ida and the Lamborghini's owner were free to go. When they arrived home, Jeff was waiting for them, concerned after hours of unanswered calls. Thankfully, he was used to their wild adventures, though even he admitted this was their craziest yet.

The next day's surprise birthday party went off without a hitch. Ida was thrilled and still couldn't believe she hadn't figured it out. The Lamborghini incident, however, quickly became the highlight of her 30th birthday weekend—a story she'd never forget.

CHAPTER NINETEEN

L indsey had been having a wonderful time in Arizona with her best friend, Ida, until she remembered the voicemail her mom had left the day before. Knowing it was likely an angry message, she decided to delay listening to it until Sunday, after Ida's birthday party. It seemed better to ruin her last day than let it cast a shadow over their celebration.

Lindsey's mom was a complicated woman, one who rarely expressed her true feelings directly. Much of this, Lindsey suspected, stemmed from her mom's early years. She had been thrust into the role of caretaker for her three younger sisters after their parents passed away just before her 21st birthday. The youngest, Aunt Joann, had been only 14. That experience cemented their family bond but also shaped her mother into someone who was deeply invested in control and responsibility.

As her only child, Lindsey often bore the weight of silent expectations. Weekends, for instance, were almost always reserved for family obligations. She loved her family but sometimes wished she could have her weekends to herself. Her dad, somehow, seemed exempt from this unspoken rule, but not Lindsey.

The voicemail, she assumed, was about her absence at breakfast on Saturday and her no-show at Aunt Mary's on Sunday. The problem was Lindsey hadn't told her mom she was out of town for the weekend, a detail she now regretted.

Ida was chatting away as Lindsey wrestled with thoughts of her mom. Lost in her head, Lindsey barely registered Ida handing her an extra bottle of water for her morning run. "You'll need it," Ida had said with a knowing smile. Lindsey nodded absently, laced up her running shoes, and headed out for her easy 4-mile run.

Arizona mornings in early June were no joke. At 7 a.m., the temperature was already in the mid-80s. Lindsey was grateful she only had a short run to complete.

Determined to rip off the Band-Aid, Lindsey called her mom as she started jogging. Her mother picked up on the first ring—a bad omen.

"Hi, Mom," Lindsey began cautiously.

Her mom wasted no time, launching into a grilling session about where Lindsey had been the day before. Lindsey hesitated, then admitted, "I'm in Arizona."

The silence on the other end was deafening.

"I don't even know my own daughter," her mother finally said, her voice tinged with hurt. "When you get back, we're having a long conversation."

Lindsey panicked and made a quick excuse to end the call. She hung up and focused on her run, though her thoughts were still swirling.

As the miles passed, Lindsey had a revelation. She was tired of constantly worrying about disappointing others, especially her mom. It was her life, after all, and she deserved to enjoy it. With that clarity, she refocused and finished her run strong, marveling at the strange sensation of sweating in Arizona's dry heat. It evaporated so quickly it hardly felt like she was sweating at all.

By the time she reached the 4-mile mark, Ida was waiting for her in the car, holding another bottle of water.

Ida always knew what Lindsey needed. Not only had she brought the water, but she'd also turned the run into a one-way trip, sparing Lindsey the effort of running back in the heat.

Back at the house, Lindsey showered and joined Ida for brunch. They indulged in Bloody Marys—salty, refreshing, and exactly what Lindsey needed after her run. The rest of the day was spent poolside, soaking up the sun and laughing about the weekend's adventures.

By the time Lindsey boarded her red-eye flight home, she felt recharged and ready to face whatever awaited her—including that long conversation with her mom.

CHAPTER TWENTY

It had been a few weeks since Lindsey visited Ida, and she couldn't shake the feeling that she was in a rut. Summer had arrived in full force—the birds were chirping, lawnmowers buzzing, and everyone had swapped out boots for flip-flops and short shorts. But with the heat came a nagging challenge: it was too damn hot to run outside.

Two months into her training, Lindsey found herself wishing for fall to hurry up and arrive. Her once-rigid schedule was slipping, and she knew it. She had promised herself to get up early this Sunday and knock out her eight-mile run before the sun made it unbearable. But instead, she was still in bed at 9:45 a.m., scrolling through her phone and procrastinating.

"Only eight miles," she told herself. It wasn't even a long run anymore—not really, not at this stage. She finally dragged herself up, pulled on her running gear, and laced up her shoes. As she reached for the door, though, she realized she hadn't had her usual pre-run coffee or banana. So, into the kitchen she went.

The coffee took its time brewing, and as it did, Lindsey flipped on the TV. The guide popped up. *Pretty Woman*, starting at 10 a.m. "Just a few minutes," she thought, settling onto the couch with her coffee and banana. Julia Roberts had barely met Richard Gere before Lindsey found herself an hour deep into the movie. Her feet were propped up, and somehow a bag of chips had appeared in her hands. Not a snack-sized bag, mind you—the family-sized one.

By 11:30, she realized she was still on the couch, still in her running gear, and still hadn't run those damn eight miles. "Loser," she muttered to herself, glancing at the screen and sighing. After the movie ended around 1 p.m., she figured she might as well have lunch. She made a peanut butter sandwich, wallowing in her frustration.

"Lindsey, stop this madness," she finally scolded herself. "You're not taking off these shoes until you run those eight miles."

And that was it. With her resolve firmly in place, she grabbed her water bottle and headed out.

The run was as miserable as she'd expected—hot, sticky, and slow, not helped by the chips she'd polished off earlier. But 6 pounds of sweat and 8 miles later, she made it. It wasn't her best effort, but it was done. At 3:30 in the afternoon, the day felt wasted, but she also felt accomplished. She had set out to run, and despite her procrastination, she did it.

Her satisfaction quickly turned to panic as she remembered she was supposed to be at her parents' house for a barbecue—an hour ago. She bolted into the shower, quickly pulled her wet hair into a bun, and slipped into an old sundress.

The dress was loose—really loose. Lindsey stared at herself in the mirror, surprised. Had she really lost that much weight? She hadn't even noticed. Running had shifted her focus so completely that she no longer obsessed over how she looked in her clothes. It was a revelation: her mind had finally let go of one of her most self-defeating habits.

As she rushed out the door, Lindsey felt hopeful. If she could conquer her inner critic, maybe—just maybe—she could find the courage to stand up to her mother, too.

CHAPTER TWENTY-ONE

The last few weeks had been a bit tumultuous for Lindsey regarding her mother. When she returned from Arizona, her mother had been cold toward her. Lindsey managed to have a brief, restrained conversation, avoiding the deeper issues, and promised to notify her mother if she ever went out of town without letting her know again. Around her mother, Lindsey always felt small, as though she lost her voice the moment her mother entered her space.

Lindsey had made it to all the required family gatherings over the past few weeks, but today she faced a hiccup. She was over two hours late to the family barbecue and was scrambling to figure out how to get back in her mother's good graces.

As she pulled up to the house, she remembered she was supposed to bring a salad. She silently cursed herself, thinking she truly was a terrible daughter. Spotting some of her cousins, she decided to head over to them, trying to mask her tardiness. Everyone seemed to be enjoying the hot, sunny day. Her dad was at the grill, expertly cooking chicken, ribs, and hamburgers. He really was a great griller.

Walking over to the table with all the side dishes, Lindsey

noticed there were already four other types of salads. Relieved, she realized no one would even notice that she hadn't brought one. That was one advantage of having lots of cousins, aunts, and uncles — there was always an abundance of food.

Aunt Joann came over immediately, complimenting Lindsey on her dress and how great she looked. Lindsey took the opportunity to ask about her mother's mood, hoping to gauge the situation. As usual, Joann downplayed any tension, brushing it off as no big deal. Still, Lindsey knew her mother would bring it up at the right moment, but for now, it was a relief to know her aunt wasn't bothered by her lateness.

After eating a plate of food and sipping on a couple of hard lemonades, Lindsey finally summoned the courage to approach her mother. Her mother was busy restocking drinks in the cooler and, upon seeing Lindsey, sighed audibly. Lindsey apologized for being late, explaining that she had an eight-mile run planned earlier in the day but had struggled to muster the energy until much later. The delay had thrown off her timing for the barbecue. Her mother seemed curious and asked if her struggles with running were because of her.

Lindsey didn't need to say anything; her mother pulled her into a hug. The gesture surprised Lindsey, and she realized she might be her own worst critic. Maybe, she thought, if she simply told her mother that she needed more time to focus on herself, her mother would finally understand. For now, though, the hug was enough, and Lindsey silently vowed to start speaking up for herself more in the future.

The rest of the afternoon was enjoyable, and Lindsey was glad she had made it, even if she was late. The day served as a reminder that it was better to show up late than not at all.

CHAPTER TWENTY-TWO

I t was another Friday and another long run as the calendar flipped to August. This time, Lindsey was fully prepared with sugar energy packets, a granola bar, electrolyte drinks, and water. She set out for her 16-mile run, the routine all too familiar. The weather started out slightly warm, and as the sun rose, the blacktop trail began to heat up. By mile 8, the phantom knee pain made its predictable appearance, something Lindsey now considered a trusted companion. Her running belt was loaded with gear that shook and rattled with every stride, rubbing against her skin in all the wrong ways.

Along the way, Lindsey realized that somewhere back at the turnaround point, she had lost her water bottle. She couldn't believe it. How could she not have heard the clunk of it falling? Sometimes, she amazed herself with how easily she could tune out the world around her, running for miles without realizing it. She was down to only half a bottle of electrolytes, and with four miles still ahead, the heat was going to drain that quickly. She started rationing her sips to half a mouthful at a time, but that only made her crave more.

At last, Lindsey reached the street that was just over a mile from home. She told herself she could make it, but in the next breath, she felt like she might collapse. She decided to listen to the second thought and began searching for any water source she could find. Then, she spotted a hose on a front lawn. The lawn was newly landscaped, with flowers blooming in bright colors. The hose had a spray nozzle attached, and it was dripping, suggesting it had been left on.

Lindsey's eyes lit up. This was her saving grace—a water source. She grabbed the hose and started drinking, managing to get more water on her face than in her mouth. The water pressure was intense, so she adjusted the nozzle, trying to soften the flow. As she gulped down the refreshing liquid, she noticed someone walking toward her, giving her a puzzled look. The sun was so bright that it took a moment for her to realize who it was.

It was the hot married guy who lived down the street. He smiled and laughed, and Lindsey couldn't help but laugh too, knowing she must look ridiculous—drenched in water, slurping from a garden hose.

He introduced himself as John and explained that he actually lived in that house, not across the street. He joked that his hose was available for runners of all shapes and sizes for a modest $15 per soak. The back-and-forth banter was filled with sarcasm, and Lindsey found herself laughing along. She thanked him profusely for the free "introductory soak" and said she might take him up on the $15 offer in the future before continuing on her run.

As she continued her final mile, Lindsey couldn't stop thinking about John. She wondered if she could get to know him better, maybe by stopping by his house the next time he was outside. Perhaps losing her water bottle hadn't been such a bad thing after all. She finished her longest run ever, 16 miles, and couldn't help but feel proud. Her treadmill was going to get a high-five from her today.

CHAPTER TWENTY-THREE

It had been a pretty fun week at work for Lindsey. She had just earned top sales for last month and, as a result, was chosen along with two of her colleagues to travel to Toronto for an all-expense-paid conference for sales executives.

Naturally, this victory was a perfect excuse for some of her coworkers to target her for their office shenanigans—a workplace norm that always seemed to strike when she least expected it. Lindsey had returned from lunch one day to find her entire cubicle completely barcoded with "property of" stickers. It was pretty hilarious. Even her sweater and pens were tagged with inventory barcodes. Whoever was behind this prank had really gone all out "inventorying" her office.

Brad, who had also earned a spot on the Toronto trip, stopped by to witness the prank. Mark wandered over too, looking for a bit of consolation after just missing the sales cutoff. It was during this mix of adulation and encouragement that Lindsey asked if they were free a week from Friday morning. She had a long run scheduled, eighteen miles, and invited them to join her.

Mark was a runner, though not one for organized races,

while Brad preferred his skateboard whenever he had the chance. Still, Lindsey, feeling a bit nervous about the upcoming distance, wondered if either of them might be willing to run part of it with her—either the outbound or return leg, each stretching nine miles.

She had a 16-mile run planned for tomorrow, but the thought of next week's 18 miles was starting to freak her out. Mark and Brad immediately started strategizing who would accompany her on which part of the run. This brought Lindsey so much relief. She wouldn't have to run alone next week. Brad agreed to skateboard the first 9 miles with her, and Mark would run the second half, even though he had never done 9 miles before. If he was slow, it wouldn't matter because she would be too, given that it would be her final 9 miles.

Meg, another winner of the Toronto trip, wandered over to see the prank and struck up a conversation about downloading books as a way to distract Lindsey on her run. Mark suggested podcasts instead, saying they were shorter and less demanding to follow. Lindsey had never considered either option, as she usually only listened to music during her runs. But the idea of downloading something different seemed intriguing. She made a mental note to try both books and podcasts on her 16-mile run on Friday.

The rest of the day at the office was filled with silliness, as more and more people were trying to leave early in the last few weeks of August. It was hard to keep salespeople in the office, especially on nice days like this. Lindsey was part of that crowd, grabbing her work bag—also barcoded—and escaping the office as quickly as she could.

CHAPTER TWENTY-FOUR

Early Friday morning, Lindsey drove over to the beginning of the wooded park where bikers, hikers, and runners all convened in the area. She figured the 2-mile run to the park would not be fun coming back from, so she cut that part out of her 16-mile route and decided to start the route at the beginning of the woods.

Today was going to be a hot one, and she figured that with all the trees, it would be way more tolerable. The bathrooms and water fountains at the entrance would be a welcome sight as well. Lindsey loaded up her items and attached them to her running belt. She got her phone out and was deciding what to listen to when her downloaded book started to play. Well, she figured that was a sign, and she hooked up her earbuds and off she went on her 16-mile run.

This book was all about a sniper who had gone rogue. It was narrated by a man and a woman, and they were fantastic. Lindsey was so into this book. It was as if she was part of what the sniper was going through. At times, she looked up and saw others pass by and continued running her pace, getting caught up in the treacherous life of the sniper and his efforts to prove his innocence.

She was having a really good run. The shade was helping keep her cool, and the book was keeping her mind occupied. Overall, she was in pretty good spirits. She passed mile 12 and continued deep into the storyline of the book. At mile 15, she looked up and realized she had no idea where she was heading. All the trees looked the same, and now she was seeing a mountain biker coming her way. How did she get on the mountain bike trail, she asked herself. Crap, this book was so good she was now totally lost. She stepped off the trail so she wouldn't get run over and started to look at her GPS. Her phone had no service. She was completely lost in the woods with no cell service.

Lindsey circled back and started to walk a bit on the mountain bike trail as she came up on her 16 miles of running being tracked on her phone. She was done with her run but had no idea how to get back to the parking lot. Up ahead came another biker, and she would try to see if that person would help guide her back to the entrance.

The mountain biker slowed his pace down to try to pass her, and they both realized they knew each other. It was John, that guy she was interested in. He stopped his bike and asked her how she was doing.

Lindsey admitted she was totally lost and had no cell service. John got off his bike and started to walk with her, showing her how to get back to the lot. He smelled really nice for a guy biking, and she was wondering how stinky she was at this very moment.

John didn't say much on the walk back, but he was insistent on walking her all the way back, so she felt like that was a good sign. Lindsey filled him in on the book she was listening to, and they seemed to get a little more at ease with each other. This guy definitely had potential, Lindsey thought to herself, and she was hoping he would ask her out.

John was impressed that she had run 16 miles already as they filled each other in on their planned days. He said by the time she would be back at the lot, she would have 18 miles clocked. John did this 10-mile ride a lot and knew exactly where the 2, 5, and 8-mile markers were.

As Lindsey got in sight of her car, John hopped back on his bike and was playing with his gears. There was a nervous energy between the both of them, and Lindsey blurted out that she would love to get dinner with him sometime. John nodded and said he was free that evening.

Lindsey mentioned that she usually grabs drinks with her coworkers on Friday but that she could bail out after one and then have dinner. John surprised her and said he could meet her at the place where she was going, and they could have dinner there. They exchanged phone numbers, and off John went back down the trails with his mountain bike.

A guy she likes meeting her coworkers. This sounded like a bad idea, but before she knew it, she was agreeing to the date. The date that was going to be incredible or go down in spectacular flames.

CHAPTER TWENTY-FIVE

Friday work calls were pretty mild, as even the distributors were taking vacations in August. Lindsey now had too much time on her hands before she met up with the gang for after-work drinks and a date with John.

Clothes of various colors were strewn all over Mr. Treadmill. Lindsey had tried them all on, and putting them back on hangers seemed like such a chore. Nothing was working. She was trying too hard. She realized that having too much time was doing the opposite of helping.

Ida managed to call her just at the perfect moment of her despair. She had Lindsey FaceTime her and try on outfits while Ida organized just the right look. Ida pointed out that her clothes were getting big and that a shopping spree in the future was needed, even via video. Lindsey missed having her bestie in town but was so grateful that video chatting worked almost as well.

Lindsey headed out the door to meet up with everyone and wondered if she should let them know John was coming or wait until they were surprised. She thought the latter would be more fun and that the group wouldn't have time to grill her with questions.

At the outdoor patioed area, Lindsey saw Mark, Mark's girlfriend, Meg and her husband, and Brad with his partner, all hanging out with drinks in hand. Lindsey never noticed that each one of them was coupled up until now. Usually, one person didn't have their significant other with them, or there were other people from her company there. This seemed more unusual, considering she invited John to join and then have dinner.

Lindsey decided on a margarita since, after a long run, they were just the perfect amount of salt needed. As she waited for her drink, Brad pointed out that she was dressed to torture the single guys today. Lindsey mentioned that Ida got her dressed, and they all agreed Ida had style and taste.

As they were commenting on her outfit choice, John showed up and walked over to the group. Lindsey had her back to him, but she could feel his energy coming up behind her. The group got quiet, and Lindsey knew she was smart not to tell them. This was going to be fun. They would be dying to know all about him, and they would have to wait until another day to find out the backstory.

John greeted the group by shaking a few of their hands and touched Lindsey's shoulder in the most loving way. Lindsey was toast. She lost her voice for a moment and then asked him to sit down.

John was relaxed around the group, and Lindsey watched him as he comfortably listened to the waitress give him the beer list on tap. John went with a funny-named IPA, and the group started laughing.

This was so natural, and Lindsey thought at this point she should throw the whole kitchen sink at him. So, she started being more herself, as it was hard to be anything else around this group, or else they would call her out on it.

The night was turning out to be a fun ending to her great week. John thanked the group for letting him join and asked if he could steal Lindsey away for a dinner with just the two of them. Lindsey was impressed that he managed to get them to agree to leave them alone, and off they went to a table indoors where they proceeded to have dinner, just the two of them.

It was a nice dinner that continued the storyline of their family upbringing and what they did for work. Lindsey brought up the first meeting with the woman across the street from John, and they laughed at how mixed-up their stories were about each other. John admitted to seeing Lindsey on many occasions run by his home since his kitchen was at the front of the house. He even teased her about the hose incident.

The date was going really well, and since Lindsey had to get up early to meet her dad for breakfast in the morning, she said goodbye to him in the parking lot. John leaned down for an awkward kiss that turned into a makeout kiss that turned into a don't-want-to-leave-the-parking-lot kiss. It was the perfect kiss to make them both want more.

CHAPTER TWENTY-SIX

I t's the morning of the 18-mile run. Lindsey waits for Brad at the running spot they had planned the week prior. He's running late, as his partner, Thomas, is always late when dropping him off. Lindsey tries not to get upset because she knows Brad and Thomas are doing her a favor. She checks her fuel, drinks, and re-ties her shoelaces to prevent shin splints like the running book advises, and waits.

As she waits, Lindsey thinks about John and their other meetings that week. He met her for lunch one day after she had finished a sales visit, and he came out to see her when she ran by his house one morning. They've yet to see each other's homes, and while they are taking it slow, the chemistry between them is undeniable. Lindsey likes the pace but knows that at some point, she'll want to tear off his clothes. For now, she's content with keeping things light, even though she senses they both could get serious quickly.

Brad shows up and they start off at a great pace. Brad is impressively performing tricks on his skateboard while keeping up with her running speed. But the clicking of the wheels starts to get on Lindsey's nerves, so she turns up the volume on her headphones. A mile later, Brad starts grilling her about John. Crap, she has no choice but to tell him bits and pieces about her run-ins with John. Brad seems satisfied, but by mile 6, Lindsey is ready to tell Brad to go ahead. The clicking of the skateboard wheels is driving her crazy, and she can feel herself getting testy. Even Brad notices and comments that she seems irritated.

Lindsey doesn't understand why she's so grumpy. Everything is bugging her. Her bright pink shoes look dingy and gray, and she's over the training. Today is the day it hits her. They finally reach mile 9, where Mark is waiting to run the second half of the route with Lindsey. Brad takes the car and heads back to the start to meet them later.

Lindsey is relieved to be rid of Brad's skateboard and runs off with Mark. Mark is in a chipper mood, but Lindsey can't help but knock him down a peg. She doesn't mean to be rude, but Mark's upbeat attitude grates on her. He tries to change the subject and starts asking about John. Lindsey regrets not telling them about John earlier, and now she's stuck retelling the story while in a bad mood.

By mile 16, Lindsey can't take it anymore and decides to push ahead. Mark has slowed down, and Lindsey just wants to be done. She tells him she'll see him at the car and takes off, leaving him behind. She knows it's rude, but she's at mile 16 and just wants this whole run over with.

Lindsey finishes the run and sees Brad waiting by her car with Mark's car. He cheers her on as she hurries to finish, and she immediately collapses onto the hood of her car. Mark is right behind her, and when he finishes, he mentions that he gave her space during the last two miles, knowing she was in a mood.

Lindsey thanks them both profusely, feeling guilty for not being the best company, but they were understanding. She says her goodbyes, gets in her car, and then realizes her period has started. No wonder she was in such a bad mood.

CHAPTER TWENTY-SEVEN

L indsey's 18-mile run had clearly taken its toll, and the start of her period didn't help either. After struggling through the run and feeling off, she made the decision to cancel plans with her friends the previous night. This morning, there was no way she was going to meet her parents for breakfast at the diner. All she wanted was to stay in bed and rest. She was realizing she might have been dehydrated, too, as she drank a bunch of water before stubbing her toe on the way back to bed.

She was still planning to meet John later at his place, but even that seemed like too much. Instead, Lindsey decided to take the day for herself. She called her mom and explained that she wasn't feeling up to breakfast and needed some self-care. Her mom was a little surprised by the term "self-care," but she wished her well, which made Lindsey appreciate the baby steps her mom was taking in understanding her.

It was a moment of self-realization for Lindsey as she thought about how much of her life she had been pushing and trying to live up to other people's expectations. Today, though, she needed to focus on herself. She pulled the blinds down and drifted off to sleep for a few more hours. When she woke up, she felt rejuvenated and made herself a big breakfast, more like lunch, and savored the lazy Saturday with a third cup of coffee. It was magical—just the time she needed.

Lindsey sent a message to John, letting him know she could only stop by for an hour later, but she was still feeling a bit off and didn't really feel like getting dressed. John was under- standing and offered to reschedule for another day or even the next day. To her surprise, Lindsey said yes to rescheduling for tomorrow. She was going to stay in her pajamas, relax, and enjoy some quality time just for herself. It felt liberating and wonderful, and Lindsey couldn't help but smile, knowing she was finally putting herself first.

CHAPTER TWENTY-EIGHT

Things were getting pretty heated between John and Lindsey. She managed to see him a few times and hang out at his home. He had a wonderful house, and she understood how he spent so much time looking out on the street of his neighborhood. It really was ingenious to have the kitchen at the front of the house. All that time spent cooking and cleaning—at least you had something to look at if you had the windows open.

Since the TV area was at the back of the house, it was much more private and intimate. They had a couple of moments on his couch where it could have gone further, but both of them slowed it down. Lindsey was on her cycle, and she wanted her first time with him to be planned after a nice evening and/or date.

The upcoming weekend included Labor Day, and her 20-miler was planned for Friday. It was the final long run before the marathon. She was going to do her run later in the day as she had a bunch of work commitments during the day before the long weekend. It was better to get it over with on Friday and have the rest of her weekend to relax and relish in her hardest run being complete.

The following weeks after would be only 13 and 8 miles before the race of 26.2 miles. She was hoping that this would be "the weekend" to have sex. She tried to keep it casual at his house Thursday night and headed home with plans that the long weekend would be spent with him. She was lucky that she had no family commitments for the weekend either, as her mother and father were going up north to Aunt Theresa's cottage. It was already starting out to be an epic weekend.

She drove home and called Ida when she got there. Ida filled her in on her plans for her wedding and her dress shopping idea for marathon weekend. Ida was flying in for the marathon and thought that would be the perfect time to go dress shopping for her and for Lindsey as she was her maid of honor in the wedding. Her parents still lived in town, and she would need to invite the rest of her family to the outing as well. Lindsey caught her up on the John situation, and Ida was placing bets on which day Lindsey would cave in to her sexual desires. She was right. Lindsey was about to explode at any minute. She was so attracted to him, and every day she spent with him, it just got more and more intense.

This month of September was going to be spectacular—John, Ida visiting, and the marathon. She just needed to get through this 20-mile run tomorrow. She pulled out her brand new red running shoes and pulled off the tags. She had tried to buy the same hot pink ones when she went to the running store this week, but there were none. The stupid shoe company already had the next models out, and she was forced to pick between red and grey/turquoise. It was time to retire her hot pink shoes as they were literally falling apart. Here's hoping the red shoes helped her with tomorrow's run.

CHAPTER TWENTY-NINE

The 20-miler loomed over Lindsey's Friday brain. She just wanted to get through the work stuff and get running. Of course, it was one of those workdays where she was stuck putting out fires. She never understood why cell phone companies launched new phones on a holiday weekend. Most people were heading out of town, and those stuck in town were in a bad mood. Add the fact that they only sent a small amount of inventory, and voila, you had instant fires.

She didn't start her 20-mile run until 4 p.m., but she figured it was better late today than tomorrow. It was still pretty warm, so she drove her car to the wooded park again and parked. She gathered her gear, slipped on her new red shoes, and started the long run. She began with a podcast or two, figuring they would distract her less than a book. She switched it up to music between miles 8 and 12. Around mile 13, she was surprised she was doing pretty well and turned off all the noise to take in the beauty of the trees and the long run on a long weekend. She felt in sync with herself. Her body, her mind, and her soul were all together on this adventure.

She got a little teary-eyed thinking of the past 4 months and her first race to where she was now. It was incredible to know that she could do it. It made her feel that she could do almost anything.

She was starting to say no to things she didn't want to do. She was listening to her inner voice more. She was realizing she was more capable than she had ever imagined. Running was really great therapy. Three hours into the run, she knew she could do it. At the perfect moment, John called to check in and see if she was done yet. She told him that she got a late start and probably wouldn't be done for another hour. He asked where she was, and she said she would call him after the run.

The next hour was dusk. She hadn't even realized that the days were getting shorter. She hurried up her pace as the woods started to get darker. Was she going to make it back to the parking lot with light still left in the day? She pulled out her cell phone and turned on her flashlight. She only had 18 percent battery life left. Here's hoping she would make it out in time. She couldn't help but laugh at her stupidity and the fact that she couldn't see two feet in front of her. She had to slow down because she couldn't even see. Would the last two miles be the death of her? She started to walk so she wouldn't trip, and up ahead, she saw a bike light coming her way. Who would be out here starting their ride at this time, she thought to herself, and then it clicked. It was John. He was coming to rescue her.

He saw her and lit up the rest of her run back to the car. She was elated. She managed to finish her 20-miler with John by her side. This immediately put her over the top. She was on a mission to get laid, and no one was going to stop her now—not even herself. She started to make out with him against the car. Their hands were all over each other. He hurriedly put his bike in her SUV, and she drove expediently to her apartment. They climbed the stairs and immediately went at each other. Mr. Treadmill was the perfect object to lean against as John started to rip off her clothes. She did the same, and they ended up on the couch, fully naked.

Her body had just run 20 miles, and she was ready to go for more. She started to spread her legs and immediately realized that sex was the best stretching after a run she could ever have. She jokingly asked John to keep spreading her legs wider and wider because it felt so good, and they hadn't even had sex yet. They were laughing, stretching, and finally, things got more serious, and he focused on the task of intercourse. It was quick, but she didn't care. She was so happy and elated.

They finally got in the shower, and that's when her legs started to buckle. She had done 20 miles and John in one day. That was pretty incredible. In the shower, he held her up, and they managed to get cleaned up. She put on some clean clothes and ordered pasta with an extra side of pasta delivered. They had a wonderful evening hanging out on her couch and managed to add a round or two of more stretching as John was happy to assist in her recovery

CHAPTER THIRTY

L indsey and John had the Labor Day weekend all to themselves. Saturday started out at the diner for breakfast. Lindsey thought she would ease John into her weekend routine without her dad there to meet them. They enjoyed a big breakfast and managed to head over to the farmer's market to grab items for the weekend for a cookout they were invited to over at Brad and his partner Thomas' place.

The rest of Lindsey's gang were all out of town, so it would be mostly Thomas' friends, which would be fewer people she knew. The plans for the weekend were not set in stone, but she wanted to make sure she had something to bring just in case. As they spent time wandering and purchasing various fruits and vegetables, Lindsey looked up and saw her Aunt Joann.

Aunt Joann had a moment of amazement in her eyes, and then she coyly walked over to introduce herself to John. Of all the people Lindsey could run into when she wanted to keep the relationship quiet, Aunt Joann was the perfect one. John seemed so at ease with her aunt as they chatted and continued to shop throughout the market. They managed to find a picnic bench to sit at and continued their conversation.

The topics were wide-ranging. John got some advice on perennials for his yard next year, Lindsey went into detail on her 20-mile run she had just completed yesterday, and Aunt Joann shared why she was not up north with her sisters. It actually surprised Lindsey to hear that Aunt Joann didn't want to go so she could have the weekend all to herself. Being the baby of the family as well, John could relate and talked about his four other siblings, who were much older than him, still living on the East Coast.

They said their goodbyes, and Lindsey felt more assured that this guy was possibly the one. It was already so different from her last relationship. This one was so easy. It was like they were additions to each other, not subtractions. She was herself without worrying about his reaction. It was such a nice change in her approach to dating. Maybe all this running had really helped her find herself.

The rest of Saturday was casual, as they ended up over at John's house grilling in his backyard. Ida managed to get in on the action of the weekend, as she and Jeff FaceTimed Lindsey and John. Ida, of course, asked poignant questions, and John actually answered them all with no hesitation. That surprised Ida and, at times, left her speechless, which Lindsey thought was hilarious. Ida was hardly ever rendered speechless.

Sunday, they both went back to the park to mountain bike and run her easy run. It was perfect, as they both met back at the lot at the end of their respective workouts.

Lindsey made a bold decision to go to Brad's party, even though she didn't know that many people, and took John with her. It ended up being a fantastic, over-the-top party. She instantly made new friends as John and she were the only straight couple. That evening, they both vowed to try more new things.

A revelation they both realized during that weekend was that they didn't venture out much past their comfort zone. So, on Labor Day, they were going to try axe throwing at the new restaurant in town and possibly the music festival as well.

It was a weekend of firsts. Lindsey was really coming into her own, and John was opening up as his own person without family dictating his life. It was becoming an exciting adventure, one that neither of them wanted to let go.

CHAPTER THIRTY-ONE

The short week after the holiday proved to be crazy. Lindsey was now juggling training for a marathon, work, family, and John. She needed something to give. The good news was that her runs were shorter for the next few weeks as she was wrapping up her training, but work was getting crazier since the fourth quarter was the busiest for phone sales. Family was constant with the commitments on the weekends, and John... John was new to this equation, and Lindsey wanted that time with him to be more.

Lindsey managed to call her mother in the middle of the week to let her know that she couldn't make it on Sunday for baking with the aunts. Lindsey didn't even worry about what her mother thought or what her response would be—a first for her.

She scheduled sleepovers with John on Wednesday and Saturday, even though she wanted more, and continued her runs on Tuesday, Thursday, and Friday. Work, however, was demanding more of her time, so she gave herself some evenings to relax alone, which included Sunday nights. This would have to do for now.

The following week was her trip to Toronto, and that was going to mess up her schedule. Life was getting messier and more fun. Lindsey just needed to organize her life like a marathon schedule—with planned days off for fun.

On one of her evenings off from everyone, Lindsey managed a shopping spree. She loved shopping for others but rarely shopped for herself. Ida was the perfect friend to remind Lindsey that she was important too—and that how you look on the outside matters. It was so nice to have an evening with Ida on the phone, helping her coordinate new outfits for her upcoming trip and the fall season. Lindsey was loving the changes in her body and confidence.

Before, Lindsey would just throw on clothes. Now, she was carefully deciding what felt good on her and what made her feel like the real her. She realized that green was becoming her favorite color, as much of the wardrobe she was buying had green in it.

Lindsey also decided that week to cut her long hair into a more manageable style that could still hold a ponytail. She managed to get a hair appointment on Friday thanks to a cancellation, and her lucky streak continued. Everything was coming together in her life. She was excited for her date and overnight stay with John on Saturday, and now she had a new hairstyle and clothes to match her excitement. She was truly enjoying her newfound life and how it felt to love.

CHAPTER THIRTY-TWO

In the past, the getaway conference to Toronto would have been a welcomed sight. Lindsey, however, had so much going on, and the week away was going to add to that chaos. She packed her running gear, new work clothes, and her heart and Ubered to the train station to meet Meg and Brad.

The two were perfect traveling companions. It was too bad Mark just missed getting invited; then the gang would have had even more fun. Brad already had cappuccinos in hand, and the astonished looks from the two told Lindsey she had dressed for success.

The silly banter went back and forth as Brad was good at making a big deal about someone's attire, and Lindsey was loving every minute of it. Each of them grabbed their seats and hunkered down with their cappuccinos for the ride to Toronto. The four hours allowed Lindsey to get work emails handled and a little back-and-forth texting with John.

John was busy at work too, and he was diving into his work even more this week with her being gone. The few days prior were a little tense with them as they juggled their independent lives and how they would merge together. She knew she was the one who was creating the drama with her insecurities. She just had to figure out how and why.

When she let go when she ran, things always worked out. Maybe this week she could figure out how to let go with John and see what happens. Her new mantra would be to let go, and work was already proving to be testing that mantra as 42 more emails showed up in her inbox.

The rest of the train ride gave her the perfect amount of time to get work organized and sign off for the next three days. The conference was full of guest speakers that Lindsey was looking forward to hearing from, and a couple of fun day/evening trips were planned by her company.

She sent John a message at the end of her train ride, checking in and asking him about next week's plans, and got off the train heading to the hotel and conference center. Brad was already in rare form and was a great distraction as they waited for their cab ride. He proceeded to give a hilarious rundown of his clients' dramas they were experiencing and how he was prepared to fix them all in the most unusual and crazy way. Lindsey thought he really should look into being a stand-up comic.

Meg was the organized one of the bunch, and she already had their itinerary out and was circling the fun activities she thought all of them would like to do. One activity was a hot air balloon ride. Lindsey wasn't so sure about that, but it was a couple of days away, and she could ponder that at least for now.

Their taxi pulled up, and off they went, each of them on work calls trying to wrap up as many client issues as possible. Lindsey was surprised one of them managed to give directions to the cab driver as they smoothly arrived at the hotel with everyone still on their calls. At a moment's time, they all ended their phone calls and hopped out of the vehicle to arrange their luggage at the bellhop.

The entrance to the hotel was grand and elegant. Lindsey

wished John would have been able to come here, as she was already thinking of a future trip planned, and this hotel would be at the top of her list. She looked down at her phone, and John still hadn't texted her back about next week. She tried not to make a big deal as it was only an hour ago she sent the text, but the insecure thoughts were starting to creep in.

Each of them left their bags with check-in and headed to the adjacent convention center to the first session of the week, a renowned motivational speaker. It was a great start to her week. This speaker was so amazing, Lindsey wanted to buy anything he was selling. She was already including some of his talking points into her future sales pitches and was feeling inspired.

Lunch was catered in a different space of the conference hall. Lindsey checked her phone again, and still no text. This was starting to get ridiculous. Was there something in her text that he misunderstood? Was she overthinking it? Meg chimed in and said to not worry and just let John be for the day. Her advice was good, but it still didn't calm her mind.

She was starting to go down dark thought paths, and the lunch conversation was becoming background noise to her thoughts. It was time to check into her hotel room and get a run in before the night's fun activities. Lindsey thought maybe that would help her get out of her head.

Lindsey used her newfound sales pitch ideas to get an upgrade to her hotel room and was already starting to release some of those repetitive thoughts. Her tactics landed her a mini-suite that was both elegant and overlooked the city. She checked out all the amenities and had her eye on the jacuzzi tub after her short run.

Lindsey got her running gear together and started running out in the vibrant city streets. She ran through a park and over to the harbor. Lindsey had a moment of clarity during that run. Whatever was going to happen with John was going to happen. He was either going to be with her for the long run or not. What was the use of worrying about what was already going to happen? The only thing she could control was herself and her thoughts. So what was the use in worrying about something that was already going to happen?

Good or bad, it made no difference except the in-between thoughts she created in her mind that weren't real. They were all made up because she actually didn't know what really was going on with John. She could only see right in front of her on her run and what was happening in the present moment. Wow, the present moment was fantastic. She realized Toronto was such a pretty place to run in. She took her time and ended up stopping at the waterfront for a bit and watching the boats go by on Lake Ontario.

She finished her run thinking about her future soak in the tub and headed back to the elevators, where she ran into Meg, who was heading back up to her room. Meg found out that Lindsey managed to get a mini-suite, and it needed a key to get up to that floor. Meg instantly called Brad, who decided that a cocktail hour before dinner should be had in her suite. Lindsey agreed and said she would meet them on their floor later to key them up to her floor.

It was looking to be a magical night, and the jacuzzi tub was just the beginning.

CHAPTER THIRTY-THREE

The evening cocktail hour at Lindsey's mini-suite was revealing. Each of them shared their relationship struggles and successes. There was candid discussion about Lindsey's ex who Meg and Brad could finally talk about since they weren't dating anymore. Both were in agreement that Lindsey was way more timid around him. Glasses of wine were poured and the subject of John was brought up by Lindsey. They were careful not to elaborate or agree with Lindsey on the situation of not getting a text back from John. They knew being in long term relationships how miscommunication can happen. They instead pointed out how Lindsey was truly herself around him and that was a good thing.

Dinner was down in the banquet hall with trapeze artists as the main attraction. Lindsey decided to let the text thing go. It had been 7 hours since she sent the text but now she decided she was finally going to stop worrying. Being present was going to be her main focus. She put her phone on silent and placed it back in her purse to enjoy the evening.

Meg finally got Lindsey to agree to the hot air balloon ride. The only problem was that they finalized their decision making a little late and the only slot available was at sunrise the following day. They called it early since they had to meet the driver at 5 a.m. and headed back to their respective rooms.

The next day came way too soon and Lindsey was questioning her decision making as it was 4:45 a.m. and she had to hurry up and put on some clothes for the morning adventure. She raced downstairs and got into the vehicle waiting for the group to drive to the departure area. The group was quiet on the way to the balloon and Lindsey was thankful for that.

They arrived at their destination 30 minutes later and hopped out of the transport vehicle. It was only then that Lindsey remembered she left her purse and phone back at the hotel. It was too late to go back, she would just have to have her friends take pictures of the experience.

The balloons were getting inflated as they stood around in the dark field, each of them in a sleepy haze. The driver of the balloon that Meg, Brad and Lindsey were going to be in was an interesting character. He already was mentioning that he used to be the 2nd best hot air balloon operator but now he was the finally the best. He was waiting for them to take the bait and they did. He then proceeded to mention the previous best operator went down with his balloon. He was trying to be funny but it only made Lindsey start regretting her decision.

They started to ascend up to 1000 feet and all three of them held their breaths for a minute. The sun started to rise and it was truly incredible. The other 7 balloons started to join them. They looked so colorful dispersed all over the sky. The balloons each went down a bit into the tips of the trees and it was as if they were all walking on clouds. It was so quiet, they could hear the animals all around. The operator took them over the lake for a brief minute and circled back towards land where morning was becoming more apparent with the sun rising to its full potential. The whole trip lasted an hour and Lindsey was hoping that Brad and Meg's pictures were capturing this breathtaking experience.

They landed quietly and effortlessly and headed over to a table filled with breakfast items and champagne. What a perfect start to the morning Lindsey thought, and relished in the banquet of food and beverages.

They got back to the hotel around 11 a.m. with the next session of speakers starting at 1 p.m. Lindsey had plenty of time to go back to her room and get situated for the day and hopefully to preview Brad and Meg's pictures of the ride they conveniently texted to her phone.

Lindsey got back to her room and immediately checked her phone that was left plugged into the wall. Lindsey's phone was filled with missed calls and texts. She had 3 missed calls and a few voicemails from her mother, one missed call from Aunt Joann, 2 missed calls from John and about 15 text messages from John as well as the photos from this morning's hot air balloon ride.

Who to check first she thought to herself. She scrolled down to John's texts and the first few were confusing. Test, test, test, was all it read. She had no idea what that meant. Then the 4th text was that he got a new work phone and all the texts weren't showing up and he wasn't sure if I sent any or called. Then there were a few random texts saying he missed me and then the last text was that he would wait for my call and that his phone number was now working as it wasn't for most of the previous day due to the whole company conversion of phone systems.

So John wasn't avoiding her she thought. All those wasted thoughts on repeat in her head. She was vowing to never let that control her longer than a few minutes ever again and called John back. It was a wonderful phone call as Lindsey recanted her morning ride in the trees and the experience of being present with John on the phone.

Her next task was to check her voicemails. Her mother's

voice was more and more strained with each message left on her voicemail. Maybe this is where she got all her overthinking from, her mother. Lindsey would have to unpack that on a different day but for now she called her mother back to find out what was so urgent.

Lindsey's lovely morning quickly changed with the phone call to her mother. Aunt Theresa's husband Ned died last night on his motorcycle while they were still up north. This was devastating to the family and now she knew why her Aunt Joann called. The funeral hadn't been scheduled because Aunt Theresa was still up north and her father was driving up with her mother to help figure things out. The whole day was surreal. Lindsey was in all kinds of spaces and realized that maybe for the first time she was going to make every moment count.

CHAPTER THIRTY-FOUR

On her last day of the conference, Lindsey took a final run along the waterfront and thought of all the good times she had with her uncle growing up. She remembered the time he taught her to ski and all the times he beat her and her cousins at poker. She had a good cry on that run and felt better for it.

The past few days in Toronto were a blur for Lindsey. She found out that her Uncle Ned would be having visitation hours on Sunday, and the funeral would be on Monday. This put another wrench in her life, as she had already been away for almost four days and work was hectic enough already. Now she would be out for Monday for a funeral, and her plans with John would have to be changed. The run had helped her manage the chaos. Running was truly therapeutic, she thought.

Their afternoon train heading home on Friday wasn't leaving until 2 p.m., and everyone had someone picking them up, including Lindsey. They met at the hotel lobby bar for a quick bite and an afternoon cocktail.

Lindsey went straight to ordering a dirty martini, foregoing the quick bite. Obviously, the run had helped but not entirely. The stress of losing a loved one had finally pushed her over the edge. Meg and Brad joined in the martini drinking with an order of a cosmopolitan and a cable car, along with a few appetizers. They managed to get an additional drink ordered and consumed before heading to the train.

The four-hour train ride home ended up being a drunken debacle. They spent most of the ride in the bar car, partaking in various unconventional cocktail choices. Meg and Brad, keeping up with Lindsey's self-destructive ways, was a no-brainer—they were all good friends who knew she needed to blow off steam, even if it meant they were drinking too much.

When they got to their stop, it was all they could do to gather their belongings and get off the train before it continued on. They practically missed getting off in time, and that set off the uncontrollable giggles, which picked up steam all the way to the parking lot.

It was Friday night at 6:18 p.m., and Lindsey, Brad, and Meg were all drunk. Unfortunately, their counterparts were not. The car rides home were going to be a lot less funny, as they were each going in separate cars with their significant others.

John didn't care that Lindsey was drunk. He knew she was going through something, and the best way he could handle it was to give her a big hug. She melted right into his arms and hugged him right back. They each headed off to their cars, and Lindsey slid into the passenger seat of John's.

John grabbed Lindsey's luggage, placed it into the back of the car, and got into the driver's seat. Lindsey, in her inebriated state, told him to take her home because she was going to do things to him that were unmentionable. He wasn't exactly sure what she meant, because she proceeded to close her eyes on the car ride home.

John got Lindsey and her luggage up to her apartment, and

Lindsey awoke just long enough to salute her treadmill before walking into her bedroom and passing out. John decided to stay the night just to make sure she was okay, and when he got in bed a few hours later, after she had been sleeping for a while, Lindsey rolled over and whispered, "I love you."

CHAPTER THIRTY-FIVE

Saturday morning was a rough one for Lindsey. She was nursing a really bad hangover. Dirty martinis were now going to be banned for life. This was her second really bad experience with them, and it wrecked all her rational thinking.

She needed to get some toast in her system pronto since she hadn't eaten since yesterday at breakfast—or maybe she had something at lunch; she couldn't recall. It was a good thing she had bread in her freezer right now, and she wondered if John stayed the night or left.

She heard the door open to her apartment, and in walked John. He had a bag of McDonald's in his hand. He was bright-eyed, and she now was wondering if she had imagined things she said last night or if they really happened.

The grease of hashbrowns and a Coke worked. John assured her that that was his go-to move when he was hungover in the past, and he was right. Lindsey was starting to feel better. Their weekend plans were a little messed up, but he was there, and she was going to make the best of it.

Lindsey took a shower, cleaned herself up, and went out to

the living room to catch John up on the details of her uncle's death and the final arrangements. They shared the rest of the breakfast with each other and cuddled on the couch until Lindsey felt more like herself. The phone rang, and it was Ida, wanting to catch up on the week and what was happening with the family and the funeral.

John motioned that she should take the call as he was going to head home for a few hours, and he would be back later to see her. The call gave her a chance to really catch her breath from the week that was and to process all the wonderful feelings she was having for John. Did she dream that she said, "I love you," or did she really say it? That was something she was going to keep from Ida for now until she processed it fully.

Ida was always her rock. She had been Lindsey's witness to everything, and just hearing her voice put her at ease. It was so great that John realized that too because maybe John was just like Ida—a rock as well. Today's hangover was already yesterday's news.

CHAPTER THIRTY-SIX

Uncle Ned's funeral was filled with cousins, extended family, and strangers. It was starting to feel like a bad idea to have John there. This wasn't just her parents, but also the whole famdamily. As Lindsey entered the funeral home, she was greeted by her Aunt Mary and her husband, who immediately extended their hand to John.

It was an emotional moment seeing her mother in the distance, trying to hold up her sister through her pain. Her mom was always the one who managed everyone's affairs, and today was no different. It was like the past when her parents died; she held the family together and made it a point to keep the traditions alive. Now, her mom was doing it all over again with Aunt Theresa and her children. Some of Theresa and Ned's kids lived out of state and were in for the funeral, and many of them were staying at her mother's house. She had planned the food prep and all of the arrangements for the funeral. She really admired her mom and was starting to fear her a little less. It was another moment when Lindsey was seeing her mom in a different light—as a person, not just as a mother.

Lindsey wanted to leave John over by the couches and head

over to the front to greet her mother and aunt by herself, but John steadily held her hand and went over with her. It was such a relief because at that moment, she really didn't think she could handle walking.

The moment they convened, it was all hugs and crying. Lindsey wasn't even sure what happened or whether she even introduced him, but it didn't matter—he was still there. Even this moment didn't scare him away.

Theresa and Ned didn't have the perfect marriage, but who really did? Lindsey thought to herself. What she did really want was someone who could help her grow, not stay stagnant. The whole point of including another person in your life was to help you grow, rally around you when you are stuck, and enjoy the present. Was John really that person? He sure was starting to resemble that kind of person, and it warmed her heart.

The rest of the visitation was John getting introduced to many of her cousins, including second cousins. She joked that there would be a quiz later tonight, but he seemed unfazed— probably because he had a big family as well.

One of Lindsey's second cousins was a runner. In fact, he had run over 20 marathons, and she was eager to get any advantage to help her on her first marathon coming up in exactly one week.

At that moment, she realized her race was in exactly one week. This was the moment she started to freak out—at a funeral home, no less. With everything going on in her life, she hadn't realized the Alien Marathon was next week Sunday.

Her cousin was full of advice, some of which Lindsey was quick to take in. One thing he did differently was use fewer sugar food packets and more salt packets. He said it kept his legs from stiffening up so much toward the end of the race—a thing she noticed big time on her 20-mile run. Another good point was to do lots of leg drains after the race to keep legs from locking up. She took out her phone and jotted down all the ideas, and the panic started to kick in even more. Did she train correctly? Again, she realized her mind was not her friend, and so she took in all the faces of her family going through trauma and remembered that what was happening in front of her was the truth. It wasn't her mind. Her mind creates drama, and with the week she was about to have, she needed less drama.

CHAPTER THIRTY-SEVEN

I t was a long and exhausting weekend. Her hangover, the visitation, the unpacking, and getting the apartment ready for Ida the following weekend took a toll on her. She never got a run in on Sunday, which was her scheduled training day, and that was putting her in a mood. Everything seemed to be a mess and perfect at the same time. It was an odd combination.

The funeral this morning wasn't until 10 a.m., and Lindsey decided to get a quick two-mile run in before she showered. This wouldn't be the four-miler she planned yesterday, but at least it was something. Lindsey decided to run by John's house to get a glimpse of him in his kitchen, if he was still there. He went home yesterday after the visitation because he had a big planning meeting this morning.

Lindsey laced up her red shoes, which were breaking in nicely, gave Mr. Treadmill a quick acknowledgment tap on his handles, and headed out on her run. It was starting to get a little cooler, and Lindsey was thinking her short-sleeve shirt was a wrong choice. It was only two miles; she could manage. Her pace was a little faster since she was doing a short run, and her lungs started to warm up along with the rest of her body.

She was remembering something her cousin said yesterday about it being 20 degrees different when you are running. It was a good way to decide what to wear for the day, especially since it was getting colder in the fall months. Since it was only 52 degrees this morning, her body would feel like it was 72 degrees when it warmed up. This was still a good temp for short sleeves, she thought, and she was right. It was just the initial leaving of her apartment that was making her second-guess herself. Her body, at this moment, felt just right.

She came around the corner and up John's street she went. His light was on in the kitchen, so she decided to flash him if he was in the window. She came up to his house and stopped. He wasn't there, so she decided to call him from her phone, and he answered on the first ring. She could see him walking around in his kitchen, but he wasn't looking out the window. Then, all of a sudden, she saw him glance over, and she decided to risk it and show him her breasts. It was freeing and funny all at the same time. John just laughed and told her to take care of them until he could later that night. He was so sensual, and Lindsey could only imagine all the fun she would be having later in the evening. She just had to get through the funeral today.

Lindsey finished her quick run and attempted to find something to wear for a funeral she didn't want to attend. She called her Aunt Joann to see if she wanted to go with her over to the church. Aunt Joann was very standoffish at the visitation yesterday, and Lindsey was wondering if she was struggling more than she let on. Aunt Joann accepted the gesture, and Lindsey went over to pick her aunt up.

Joann was slightly disheveled looking, a look rarely seen by Lindsey or anyone else, for that matter. It was a bit unnerving because Joann always was put together and happy. Had this death really affected Aunt Joann?

She slowly got into the car, and Lindsey decided they both needed fancy coffees in order to make it through the service. She drove over to the drive-thru of the local coffee shop and proceeded to order coffees with extra whipped cream. It was the cream that did the trick, and Aunt Joann started to talk. She was having an existential crisis. She was at a point in her life wondering if it made sense at all and if she was really happy being alone. The death of Ned made her question all of her decision-making and, most of all, being single. Lindsey didn't really have words of advice, but she continued to listen in the parking lot of the coffee shop.

It was a special moment that she shared with her aunt, and she held her hand and comforted her with her grief. Her take-away from the death of Ned was to be more present in her life, and she shared that with Aunt Joann.

Aunt Joann just needed to figure out what part of her life she was needing to change with the news of Uncle Ned. Maybe it was nothing, but maybe it was more. Lindsey shared her fears about life and death, and when Aunt Joann was ready, maybe she would share as well.

The funeral ended up being a celebration of Ned's life. There were lots of stories being shared about Ned's poker-playing ways and his knack for teaching and instruction-giving. The focus was more about what we gained from living than what we lost. It was actually more uplifting than Lindsey thought.

The family gathered back at her mother's house for more food and storytelling. It was getting late, and Lindsey went up to her mother to let her know that she did a wonderful job cele-brating Ned's life. Her mother looked relieved, and Lindsey realized her mother also looked a bit scared. She didn't know what to do with that, so she gave her mother a quick hug and let her know she was driving Aunt Joann home.

It was odd, Lindsey thought on her drive to John's after she dropped off Joann. It was as if she was processing her trauma through her running, and her family hadn't ever processed their trauma.

It was like she was more in the energy of a parent, and her mother and aunt were more in the energy of children. It was a moment of clarity. She was becoming increasingly her authentic self, and she was content. Maybe, just maybe, she could help her family get to that space as well.

CHAPTER THIRTY-EIGHT

I t was already Tuesday, and Ida was texting with all kinds of ideas for the marathon weekend. The entire weekend, including Thursday night, was already planned. Ida was landing with her fiancé, Jeff, around 3:30 p.m. on Thursday, and John was finally going to meet her best friend. She just had to buckle down and get five days of work done in just two. Luckily, work came easy to her, and she holed herself up in her cube until her spreadsheets and reports were complete.

This was a week she told her coworkers that was off-limits to their work shenanigans. It was understood that someone could call off practical jokes during certain crazy work weeks. This gave everyone a reprieve, but she knew they would be back at it after the marathon. Lindsey would be hyper-focused on the pranks next week, she told herself, and got back to the immense job of getting things done.

At the end of the day, John called and asked if she wanted to come over to his house and stay the night and the rest of the week. Already, the back-and-forth between places was starting to get messy. Lindsey had some of her clothes at his place and some of his things at hers.

She was planning to have Ida and Jeff stay at her place, and her one-bedroom place was not ideal. She was setting up the living room for herself while they took her bedroom. The only problem was that Mr. Treadmill was taking up a lot of space in the living room, and her blowup bed was going to be tight when she set it up. If only she could get rid of that treadmill.

John suggested, since her week was so hectic, that she stay the entire week at his place and that Ida and Jeff could stay in his guest bedroom that already had an entire ensuite. This was such a grown-up experience for Lindsey. Was she ready to share her friends, his house, and all the in-betweens for an entire week?

His suggestion did make a bunch of sense, and it would be a lot easier, so she agreed. She went home, grabbed the rest of the stuff she would need for the entire week, and went over to John's for the trial week of living together.

Ida was shocked that, with all her planning, she did not have staying at John's in those plans. She laughed via video chat and wanted a tour of her ensuite that she would be staying in when she and Jeff visited. John humored her and took her out to the garage. They all laughed when she realized he was just joking, and he finally showed her room. Lindsey was already starting to feel like John was part of her, and she was part of him.

That evening, John and Lindsey set up their bedroom. Lindsey managed to hang a few items in the master closet and even got a couple of drawers to put her things away. It felt actually natural.

Lindsey loved John's home. Its contemporary style was complemented by a touch of traditional furnishings, creating a warm and inviting atmosphere. She was impressed to learn that John's older sisters had helped him choose his bedroom sets, which explained the subtle but thoughtful details that gave the space a more polished, refined look. Everything about the house felt cozy and welcoming, and Lindsey found herself genuinely happy to spend the week there. This marathon week was shaping up to be unforgettable.

CHAPTER THIRTY-NINE

Thursday morning arrived with the same excitement Lindsey used to feel on Christmas as a child. Her best friend, Ida, was coming to town, and the anticipation was electric. She woke up buzzing with energy, ready to tackle the day. John was already in the kitchen brewing coffee while Lindsey laced up her sneakers for her final pre-race run. The past few days at John's place had been unexpectedly comforting, it all felt so natural.

Grabbing a quick half-cup of coffee, Lindsey headed out into the brisk morning air. The chill reminded her of the weekend's forecast, and she started to worry about what to wear for the race. Dressing for the fluctuating temperatures was always a challenge. She steadied her breath, trying to calm her anxious thoughts. As the streetlights illuminated her path, she appreciated the quiet calm of the early morning.

Today, she chose to run without music or podcasts, letting the stillness surround her. She knew that keeping her mind steady and focused was crucial for the whirlwind ahead. The recent text message drama had taught her that her mind could be her own worst enemy if she let it.

Breathing deeply, Lindsey focused on the present moment. The cool air filled her lungs as she relaxed into her pace. She noticed the silence of the neighborhood, broken only by a few homes with lights on and one person walking their dog across the street. Otherwise, it was just her and the peaceful solitude of the morning.

When she returned to John's, she was pleasantly surprised to find breakfast ready. She hadn't thought of John as much of a cook—they usually ate out together—but he had managed to whip up omelets, bacon, and toast. The toast was the same artisanal bread they'd sampled at the farmer's market, and it was wonderful. Lindsey didn't care if the rest of the meal tasted perfect or not; the gesture alone melted her heart. No one she had dated before had ever made her breakfast. As she sat down with her refreshed cup of coffee, she couldn't help but think, *This man is a keeper.*

On her way to work, she quickly caught up with Ida to confirm where she and Jeff should be picked up at the airport. She knew work would be hectic and there would be little time to coordinate everything in between. She had originally planned to take Friday off before her Toronto trip and the funeral, but with everything so hectic, she was considering going in for a bit in the morning to make the Monday after the marathon less overwhelming. She decided to make that call after plowing through the day.

When she arrived at the office, she was greeted with a trail of chocolate-covered raisins leading from her cubicle to the bathroom. Following the trail, she found a big "Good Luck" sign taped to the bathroom door, along with a cheeky reminder to use the restroom before the race. It was her coworkers' way of wishing her well, even though pranks were supposed to be off-limits this week. Lindsey couldn't help but laugh. She decided to let it slide—they meant well, after all.

CHAPTER FORTY

Ida and Jeff landed early as Lindsey was just leaving work. Her day at work actually went pretty smoothly. After the poop joke, Lindsey got super focused and managed to get her reports and commission checks reviewed in time. She didn't need to come in on Friday like she thought she would, and her ride to the airport was the perfect amount of time to decompress for fun with her best friend.

As she pulled up to the airport, Ida was already making a scene. Her drop-dead gorgeous looks and wild personality made everyone notice. She was her best friend, and she was so lucky to have this energy in her life. Jeff was on his phone, probably on a work call, as Lindsey pulled up and parked the car. The whooping and hollering between Lindsey and Ida was contagious, as the two girls embraced, making Jeff have to end his call quickly due to the loud noise.

Jeff was such a good sport. He knew when the two of them got together, it was an octave or two louder. He just took it all in stride, and Lindsey was thankful for that. They put all their bags in the car and headed over to John's place. John was still at work and was going to meet them later at the restaurant. This restaurant was one of Ida and Lindsey's favorite places when they used to live in the same town. The Greek fare was fantastic, and they loved the saganaki. Who doesn't love cheese on fire?

Lindsey got them situated at John's and gave them a proper tour of his place. Of course, since John wasn't there to defend himself, Ida immediately started giving Lindsey ideas of what she could do to the place now that she was living there. It was funny and a little scary having Ida already think that Lindsey was living there permanently. They hung out for a bit and then headed out to meet John at the restaurant.

John was already getting them a table when they arrived. Ida took one look at John and ran over to give him a hug. John hugged her back. It was so sweet seeing the two of them in the same place, Lindsey thought. John and Jeff started chatting, and the four of them headed to their table. Ida gave everyone the rundown on the weekend plans, and Lindsey was making fun of her over-planning.

During the conversation, it came up that neither Jeff nor John had ever had saganaki, so two orders of fiery cheese had to be ordered. The girls even asked the waiter to make it dramatic as he set the cheese on fire. It was delicious and hilariously fun. Ida and Lindsey continued to order their favorites, and one by one, the guys tried them all.

The evening continued back at the house, where John was able to share in his love of building Legos with another fellow Lego enthusiast, Jeff. Ida immediately gave her a cue to Lindsey to go to a separate room, where they shared more intimate thoughts and silly banter just between themselves.

CHAPTER FORTY-ONE

Friday was the planned day to go wedding dress shopping for Ida and to try on bridesmaids' dresses. Ida already had the bridesmaids' dresses picked out online, so it was just a matter of trying on the various sizes to special order. Lindsey was looking forward to having this day with Ida, for the most part, all to herself. Jeff and John both were working, so it was a day to have girl time. Ida did need to see some of her family at some point, but she decided not to have them come while she shopped for wedding dresses. She wanted to pick out her dress all to herself with no undue influence from her family.

What she didn't mention was that she scheduled Lindsey for a wedding dress fitting too. By booking them both at the same time, she got extra time in the wedding dress shop with no one else but Lindsey, and they gave her a longer appointment time because there were two brides. The only problem was, Lindsey was not a bride, and Lindsey wasn't notified she was a bride until their drive over to the shop.

"Come on, Linds, this will be fun," Ida said as they were getting out of the car. "Just make up a wedding date and go try on dresses with me," she said quickly as she was fumbling with her purse and coat.

Lindsey was already planning on trying on bridesmaids' dresses—what was the difference if she also tried on wedding dresses? So, she agreed as they made their way into the store. She started down various aisles looking for dresses that she thought Ida would like, and then, out of nowhere, she spotted "THE DRESS." It was so princess-like and totally not her, but what the heck, she thought, why not try it on?

She and Ida spent another half hour pulling dresses out, and into the dressing room they went to try on the various brides-maids' dresses that were pulled by the employees and the wedding dresses.

The attendant was all interested in their wedding plans, and Ida was hamming it up when it came to Lindsey's. In fact, Lindsey was coming up with creative ideas for her "fake" wedding as well. It was a magical day of dress-up and make-believe. A perfect balance for a Friday afternoon with her best friend.

Ida must have tried on close to 20 dresses, and nothing. Not one dress made her want to put down a deposit and buy. Lind-sey, on the other hand, put on the first bridesmaid dress, and voila! The dress was exactly what Ida was hoping for in look and style for her wedding.

Lindsey also tried on "THE DRESS," and holy shit, it was incredible. Even Ida was surprised it looked that good on her, since it was in no way, shape, or form what Lindsey would normally gravitate toward. They both stared at each other and started laughing.

"You have to get it," Ida emphatically stated. She was right, Lindsey thought to herself. It was the most perfect dress, and she had to get it. But she wasn't even getting married, let alone engaged.

It must have been the one glass of champagne talking, as

Lindsey found herself putting a deposit on a dress that she didn't remotely need. All this time shopping, and not one dress for Ida. Lindsey, however, was now the proud owner of two dresses.

Ida ended up canceling with her family, as she still had not found a dress, and Lindsey and Ida ended up all over town, shopping the day away and enjoying each other's company.

Since they managed to evade Ida's family during the day, it was suggested that they all come over to visit her dad and step-mom, her brother, and sister-in-law at her dad's house for cock-tails. Ida gave Lindsey a look that mentioned she didn't want to stay long, and they agreed to head over there before dinner.

Jeff joined Ida over at her dad's house later that day with Lindsey. Lindsey only stayed for a bit and headed back to John's, letting Ida know that it was fine to cancel dinner plans and that she would see her later if she needed a ride back to the house.

Ida always had fun with her family, even though she would rather spend every waking minute with Lindsey. She knew it was a good idea to give her the night off to spend with her family. Lindsey was also looking forward to some alone time with John as well.

She called John and surprised him with carry-out dinner and a movie for just the two of them.

CHAPTER FORTY-TWO

With everyone back at John's house, it was scheduled on Saturday to head over to the diner to have breakfast with Lindsey's family. Aunt Mary joined them with Lindsey's dad and mom.

Of course, Ida had to keep throwing off-comment remarks about Lindsey's purchase yesterday. She and Ida couldn't believe she bought a wedding dress. Was she going to tell anyone? Absolutely not. This was to go down with the grave or until she got engaged, whichever came first.

Aunt Mary shared with the group that she just had a reiki session with a woman in town the day before. She said it helped immensely process her grief and that she was taking her sisters to see her later today, even Lindsey's mother. Lindsey's mom nodded in agreement.

The diner conversation between the group got lively, and the only thing Lindsey could focus on was that her mom was going to get a reiki treatment. A reiki treatment? This was so unlike her mother. She was not someone who tried anything new, let alone this. Maybe her marathon running was really rubbing off on her family.

Packet pickup for race day was today at the expo center. So they headed down to the center after breakfast to pick up Lindsey's numbers. The whole expo was filled with running gadgets. There was so much running stuff that it was overwhelming.

Lindsey couldn't even get through the first aisle, and she purchased a flashing glow-in-the-dark ring and bracelet for the run. She had no idea why she wanted it, but she wanted it—for the race. There were other things that she was feeling like she would need. A new running belt that had even more things that could attach to it while running—maybe she needed that as well.

She continued her crazy shopping and bought a hat, shirt, and gloves, all commemorating her first marathon. The clothing was in weird black and fluorescent designs depicting aliens all over it. Any other person would have just walked by these odd-looking designs, but the Alien marathon was no boring race. They prided themselves on over-the-top-looking designs.

There were some questioning looks from Jeff and Ida, but otherwise, they were all on board with whatever Lindsey wanted, since this was a big deal. Not one of the group had ever run a marathon, so they were already quite impressed Lindsey was running one.

They got to the end of the expo, and Lindsey picked up her race shirt and bag of goodies along with her bib number. Her number was 11716. It had her name written on the top and it was shaded in green.

Lindsey saw others had different shaded bibs as well, so she asked the volunteer what the green bib stood for. It was for runners running their first-ever marathon. Oh great, Lindsey thought, now everyone will know it's my first—how embarrassing.

There was also a booth for green bibs that was all about inspiring the runners. The group was there to encourage spectators to write a letter to their first-time marathoners to read at the end of their race. Ida, already, was grabbing the free paper and envelopes, making everyone in the group, including John, take some for their own. Lindsey was somewhat excited and scared to read what they might write.

The afternoon was enjoyable, but Lindsey couldn't help but start to get anxious. The marathon that she was training for was happening in the morning. It was less than 24 hours away. She mentioned to John that she was a bit overwhelmed, and he took her cue to gather the group up and head back to the house.

When they got back to the house, Ida mentioned that she had a playlist made up for her for the marathon. She was able to transfer the song list with the help of Jeff after a few hours of swearing. She had about five and a half hours of music carefully selected for Lindsey for the day of her race. Lindsey was so curious to see what songs were chosen, but she listened, for once, to Ida and decided she would be surprised in the morning when she was running.

Already, Lindsey was doing something different than what she had planned for the marathon. Was that a good omen or a bad omen? As the night progressed, Lindsey got out her outfit along with her green bib number and put the four pins on her shirt. She grabbed her new running belt and then thought better of it and went back to her old belt, just in case it rubbed the wrong way on her waist. She got out her new flashing neon rubber ring and bracelet and placed them by her gear. She had everything she needed except her good running socks.

She realized at that moment that those socks were still at her apartment in her dryer. Now panic set in, and Ida, with a clear head and mind, mentioned that the two of them drive over to her place and get them before dinner.

She and Ida headed over to Lindsey's place and went into the apartment. Ida immediately made fun of her place with that 1980's treadmill sitting in the middle of her living room looking like the eyesore it was. Lindsey introduced her to Mr. Treadmill and laughed along with her, stating that it was too heavy to get out of her place without a lot of help.

Ida placed a call to Jeff and had the guys come over to get it out ASAP. She was such a ball buster, Lindsey thought, and she was happy for it. Who knows how long that contraption would have sat in her living room? The guys showed up, and between the four of them, they were able to get it down to the bulk pickup dumpster at her apartment.

Lindsey grabbed her socks, and when she came back to the parking lot, it was already decided that they take two cars over to dinner since it was right around the corner. Lindsey joined John in his car as Ida drove Jeff in Lindsey's car.

As Lindsey got in the car, John immediately said he would have been happy to help move the treadmill earlier if she would have just mentioned that she wanted to get rid of it. Lindsey thought his gesture was so sweet. She realized at that moment that she needed to vocalize more of what she needed and, especially, when she needed help.

It was hard for Lindsey to ask for help. Ida just knew her so well that she didn't even need to say anything. She was going to speak up more when she was with John, and with that statement in her head, she leaned over and told John that she needed him to kiss her.

There was a bit of romantic smooching as they parked outside the restaurant. It was all Lindsey could do not to tear off his clothes in the car. Sex was definitely on the table tonight before the marathon, Lindsey thought, as they hurried up to meet up with the other couple.

It was decided that they would go to a restaurant with pasta choices, as Lindsey had heard that it was good to carb up before the marathon. Again, this was her first race, and most of what she was doing was through books and hearsay. She decided on pasta with meatballs and red sauce and their amazing garlic bread. This was the sole reason for going to this particular restaurant: their unlimited garlic bread. This was the best part of running—eating all of that bread.

They enjoyed a bottle of wine with their meal, and the rest of them ordered another drink after dinner. Lindsey thought better of it and decided that her one glass of wine was enough. John was figuring out the race course at the dinner table and mentioning that he was going to take his bike so he could get to spots quicker if need be.

Ida was putting together a list of things needed at the finish line, including two bottles of champagne and Lindsey's marathon race shirt to wear after for pictures. She was also strategizing with John what mile markers they would be at so that Lindsey could know where her friends and family would be.

They finished their planning and their drinks, paid the bill, and headed home. When they got home around 8 p.m., Lindsey decided to head to bed. The 4:30 a.m. alarm was just around the corner, and Lindsey needed as much sleep as she could.

She said goodnight to everyone and motioned for John to join her. He went with her to the bedroom, and they went straight into action. He definitely helped her stretch her legs and get her ready for the marathon. He gave her a kiss goodnight, changed into his sweats, and headed back down to the movie Ida and Jeff had just started.

Lindsey lay awake in her bed, making sure she had everything she needed. Remembering she forgot to pack salt packets, she hopped out of bed and grabbed them, placing them by her gear. That's it, she said to herself. She had everything she needed; now she just needed to find her courage for tomorrow.

CHAPTER FORTY-THREE

That 4:30 alarm came pretty quickly, and then the fear followed. Lindsey quietly got out of bed, trying not to wake John. She didn't need to leave the house until 5:30, so she wanted to at least give him an extra half hour of sleep. As she fumbled around in the dark, the light switch went on. John rolled over and whispered that her trying not to wake him up was actually waking him up. So he got up and made the coffee.

She was actually thankful for that, as she was already stressing out. She immediately put her gear on and went into the kitchen to try to get something to eat. She settled on peanut butter and toast with an apple. Her hope was that she would be able to poop before the race started. It seemed to be an important thought that continued all the way until they left the house. She wasn't able to go at the house, so the porta-potties would have to do. It was not ideal, but she had no choice.

John drove her in the dark to the starting area, where he dropped her off. He mentioned that the cheering squad would be at mile 8, so look for the group then. He kissed her goodbye and wished her good luck, checking one last time at her bib number so he could track her race.

Lindsey got out of the warm car, realizing it was much colder than she had anticipated. John grabbed one of his towels in the back seat and handed it to her. That was the perfect layer to get her through the next 45 minutes before the race started at 7 a.m. sharp.

She wandered over to the corrals at the starting gate and got into her letter. It was pretty far back since she anticipated a 12-minute mile. She actually had no idea how fast or slow she was going to run. It was a complete guess, and she ended up in letter J. This meant that A, B, C, D, and so on were all faster runners than her—or at least they lied to themselves on how fast they ran. That alone made her more nervous and second-guessing herself. She was already at the back of the race, and the race hadn't even begun.

Once she got in her section, letter J, she saw a few more green bibs and realized that many were probably feeling the same way as her. She acknowledged a few of her fellow green bibbers, and they waved back. Maybe this green bib thing was a good idea, she thought.

Still having not pooped, Lindsey moved over to the porta-potties near her corral and tried to will herself to poop as she stood near the line. Nope, nothing. She couldn't get her bodily functions to work, so she got back on the street and waited for the start.

There were a few announcements and the singing of the national anthem, and right away, the starting gun went off. The crowd was moving, and Lindsey hadn't even gotten her music set up on her phone or her earbuds in her ears—and now she had to poop.

She shimmied out of the street, trying not to get trampled, and headed over to the porta-potties again. This time, her bowels were ready to explode. Who knew that the singing of the national anthem and the starting of the race would create a release of bodily fluids? As she stood in line, she got her earbuds situated and prayed she wouldn't poop her pants.

Just in time, a stall opened, and she was in business. The explosive diarrhea made it into the toilet. Whew, Lindsey thought, that was a close one.

She hurriedly pulled up her pants and joined the corral with the letter K, since her group was already too far ahead for her with the crowd. The starting line was lit up and jamming with loud music to get the runners going. Lindsey kept walking and stopping as the group finally moved in cue to the start. Letter K was now in position as the starts were staggered. She looked up at the START sign, took a deep breath, turned on her playlist that Ida created for her race, and off she went.

CHAPTER FORTY-FOUR

Katrina and the Waves started Lindsey's playlist as she headed out past the START. It was one of Ida and Lindsey's all-time favorites and immediately put her in a good mood. It was 7:20 a.m. and pitch black dark, and she remembered that she had a glow-in-the-dark bracelet and ring that she forgot to turn on while *Walking on Sunshine* was jamming. Now, with her flashing neon jewelry, she felt she was ready to conquer the world. The crowd of runners was in good spirits, already pulling off and dropping sweaters and clothing everywhere. It was a bit of a hazard as she was running barely a half mile into the race. The pace was a little bit fast as Lindsey's nerves were the energy of the first mile. She started to feel a bit more like herself right around mile marker ONE and steadied her pace.

So far, Lindsey was enjoying the playlist and the surroundings. Her shoelaces and socks seemed to be feeling right, with just the right tightness. She started her body sensing and checked in with each part of her body, making sure they relaxed and had good form. It was still pretty dark, so she was being extra careful watching the road and its unevenness.

It was just past mile marker ONE that Lindsey started to burp up last night's garlic bread. She was now regretting the extra bread she had eaten. The burps got more and more frequent, and it wasn't especially fragrant as it came up. She could only imagine that anyone in close proximity would think she reeked of garlic. It was somewhat uncomfortable and distracting, almost to the point that she was thinking about swearing off garlic bread for the rest of her life.

She looked around on the streets and saw a band that looked not quite awake playing music up ahead. This must be the entertainment the Alien Marathon mentioned on their race map. The band was dressed in Martian-looking outfits, so they had that going for them, but their music playing wasn't up to par. Lindsey just turned up her music to drown them out and proceeded on the race route. The thought of more bands up ahead was already starting to annoy her. She tried not to think of it and continued practicing her running form and keeping her arms relaxed.

Then the thought of her buying a wedding dress popped in her head, and she daydreamed for a while on the future wedding and how she would look in that amazing dress. She even started thinking about how she would wear her hair and what color bridesmaids' dresses. She definitely wouldn't pick the champagne color dress that Ida had for her upcoming wedding. She was thinking more primary colors like blue or green. Maybe she would have a fall wedding. She would have to make sure the wedding didn't coincide with football games that her family loved, and it couldn't be too close to the holidays.

She imagined that John was there at the wedding and they were having their first dance in that amazing dress. She focused on the shoes she was wearing and whether or not they would have some sparkle on them. Yes, she definitely thought sparkle would look fabulous as they danced the waltz—no, the tango—at the wedding. Her wedding plans were getting so elaborate in her mind that when she looked up, she was at mile marker TWO.

Wow, she thought, I have only 24.2 more miles to go. She checked her pace and noticed it was already way faster than what she had planned. She was running closer to 10-minute miles. It was only 7:41 a.m., and she had already run two miles. She had only six more miles until mile eight, when she would see familiar faces. This was a good thing. She focused on her music and went back to the task of running.

Up ahead, there was the first big incline where some runners were already walking. Lindsey wasn't going to let herself walk already at mile two. She looked down at the road and focused on sending encouraging words to herself to block out the heavy breathing and burning legs she was experiencing, and randomly, a stupid song popped in her head and she began repeating it in her head over and over until she reached the top of the hill. She was having an out-of-body experience where she willed herself to do something hard, and it happened.

Heading back down the hill, Lindsey got back into the present and skipped to the next song on her playlist. She was glad no one had told her about that hill prior to the race. It was taking quite a few people down to a walking pace and dampening a few people's spirits. She was none the wiser and she was glad for it.

CHAPTER FORTY-FIVE

The sun was just beginning to rise, and the road was greeting Lindsey with a foggy mist. It was quiet for a minute as she made a left on the route, where there were few spectators. She turned down her music to hear her feet pounding on the pavement. The rhythmic pounding of her shoes was actually enjoyable as the sun started to make her eyes squint.

She couldn't have asked for better weather. It was perfect for runners— a little chilly in the morning and warming up to around 60 degrees by the end of the race. She had heard nightmare stories about races in freezing temperatures and pouring rain. She was counting her blessings that at least the weather was in her favor. She was still regretting her dinner choice, however, and wished the aftermath of garlic burps would subside. That was her own doing, and she vowed to eat bland food in the future if she ever did run another race.

The sun finally rose just as Lindsey was passing mile marker THREE. It was the first water/electrolyte station, and she was unsure whether she should drink something now or at the next mile. She decided to take a little of the electrolyte and slowed her pace down to a walk. She couldn't understand how anyone could run and drink at the same time, especially with an open cup. The other reason for walking while drinking was that she hated to have sticky hands. The stuff they gave her at the last race was full of sugar and had made her hands sticky for the rest of her race.

She also relished in the few minutes of walking. It was definitely a mind game she was playing with herself, and somehow, the little walk was making her feel better. She managed to get her cup in one of the trash cans, and in an instant, she was off running again. Already, her mind was telling her to walk a few more minutes. It was literally trying to get her to quit, and it was only mile three. She had to shake that thought and decided at the next water station she would skip it and drink from her belt instead, since it had a nozzle. She was going to one-up her mind, she thought, and turned up her music.

By now, it was full daylight, and she could see more of the people and entertainment up ahead. She saw a large blow-up spaceship that was directing the racers towards the river. This really was a weird race, she thought, and saw that there were high school cheerleaders from a local school there to cheer the runners on as well. Since Lindsey was towards the back of the runners, being letter J or K for that matter, she got the less than enthusiastic cheerleaders, as they were probably cheering for at least an hour. It was still great because it was something new to look at, and they were still cheering for you, albeit at a lower energy level. It was still motivating, and Lindsey waved to them in appreciation.

She was starting to pass a few that were already walking. She wondered if they were running the full or the half marathon. She tried not to dwell too long on those who slowed down because Lindsey might find herself in that space as well.

She looked down at her impulse-purchased blinking ring and switched it off. No need to waste the battery if it was already daylight, and she continued running. The light-up bracelet had already stopped working around mile two, so she was going to pitch it after the race. Up ahead, there was a family with signs—not her family, but it was still cool to see funny signs. One of the signs said, "Worst parade ever." Lindsey got a kick out of that and agreed. It was the worst parade ever for people having to watch runners looking frustrated, tired, walking, and sweaty. She continued to laugh about it for the next half mile. There was a couple running near her; the guy had a green bib on, and the lady had a white bib. It was his first, and who knows how many she had run. They seemed irritated with each other, as he wanted to run a bit slower than the pace she was running. There was some back-and-forth discussion about staying together and also her going ahead.

Lindsey felt glad that she was running this race by herself. It was hard enough with the mind games of running the marathon, let alone letting someone down or being worried about someone else. As they all approached mile marker FOUR, the lady in the white bib took off.

She had left her guy back with Lindsey. The two of them side by side ran for another few minutes until the guy said out loud that he was glad she left. He said she was only running the half marathon and that it was messing with his head. Lindsey gave him some encouragement as they came upon the next hydration station. He ended up stopping to get water as Lindsey continued on.

CHAPTER FORTY-SIX

Halfway between mile four and mile five, Lindsey was questioning why she was so hyper-focused on the mile markers. She had literally run a bunch of training runs, and hardly once did she struggle as much as today at miles four and five. Was it because the race had gigantic mile marker signs? She would love to give the race organizers a piece of her mind about the enormous numbered signs. She thought that in the future, they should have tiny little, barely visible markers to help the future runners run a better race. Yes, that would be an excellent suggestion, she thought.

As she was still pondering the size of the mile markers, she heard someone yelling her name. She looked up, and it was John. John was on his bike between mile four and five. How exciting, she thought, and her energy perked up. John then mentioned that he wasn't going to be at mile eight because he had to get a few more things for the finish line. He didn't elaborate, and Lindsey was in no condition to ask too many questions. She needed to keep as much energy to herself as she could. He offered to take anything that she didn't need, and she handed him her light-up ring for safekeeping. He gave a quick hug and a kiss, and off she went—Lindsey running one way and John biking the other.

Wow, what an energy booster, Lindsey thought, and she was glad to have family and friends out there cheering her on. This was definitely going to help. She cheerily ran up the road until she saw it: the large mile marker FIVE putting her back in her head again. At least she had already run five and only had a bunch more to go.

She skipped the hydration station again, and luckily, the next song on her playlist was one of the Pointer Sisters' hits from the '80s. This was an ideal running tune as it had the energy to push her and focus on running. She focused on the older gentleman up ahead, his bright green shirt with a picture on the back. He must be running in memory of someone. She couldn't quite make out the picture of the person on the shirt but gathered it was a younger person, as she was figuring out the math in her head of the deceased person's date of birth and death. Now, she couldn't help wondering how that person died and what their relationship was. What a motivated runner he was, as she followed his pace for the next mile.

She noticed another funny sign as she got to mile marker SIX that mentioned they had already run a 10k. The only problem was that it was at mile six and not two-tenths later. They had good intentions, but it was lost in translation. Lindsey was such a critic at this point in the race. She became aware that this race was making her more cynical.

She needed to have more fun. She reminded herself that it was a day just for her. All these people were clapping just for her. As she started to do this, a couple of people started yelling out her name and telling her what a great job she was doing as a first marathoner. They must have known about the green bibs, she thought, and was thankful for the encouragement. It lifted her spirits, and she kept on running.

When she got to mile marker SEVEN, she fumbled around for one of her salt packets that her cousin had suggested. She kept trying to open it as she was running, but couldn't get the packet to rip, so she ended up putting the whole salt packet in her mouth and swallowing. It would have to do, she thought, and continued running.

Up ahead, the next water station had more volunteers dressed with alien-antennae headbands. She stopped this time to get some water and walked for a few minutes. Again, her mind was trying to trick her into taking a longer break, but she willed herself to ignore it and took off running again, knowing her family was up at mile eight waiting.

Lindsey took on the next mile with such gusto. Mile marker EIGHT came into view for a brief second, but her eyes immediately went to the screaming crowd on the left. It was her mom, dad, Aunt Joann, Theresa, Mary, a few of her cousins, Jeff, and her best friend Ida. They had signs made with hilarious pictures of Lindsey blown up to a very large size. She immediately ran over to that side of the street to high-five the family and hug a few of them. It was so amazing and special that Lindsey's heart just melted.

The group was especially vivacious, and Lindsey realized they were all having champagne and Bloody Marys. Here she was running for the last hour and a half, and they were drinking her celebratory champagne. She couldn't help but laugh a little.

Ida was trying to run a bit with Lindsey, telling her that John went to get more champagne for the group since he had a bike and that they were having a marvelous time drinking and cheering on the runners. Of course, her family would be having fun—they knew how to make the best of any situation.

It was especially good to see Aunt Theresa actually smiling, since the funeral was only a week ago. Maybe Lindsey should have run in memory of her uncle, she thought, and kept running, thinking fondly of him. From a distance, she heard her family yell out that they would see her at mile fifteen, and Lindsey was happy she had another future encounter to look forward to with her wild and crazy family.

CHAPTER FORTY-SEVEN

As Lindsey ran further and further away from her family, a pain in her knee started to act up. It was that same phantom knee pain that had occurred during her training at the eight-mile mark. What was this all about? Was eight miles her limit? Did she have a limit? Was this a test?

The pain gradually started to dissipate the minute she acknowledged it. It must be psychosomatic, she thought, and began analyzing herself and why she feared running beyond eight miles. For some reason, she could wrap her head around eight miles, but anything past that made her feel anxious.

But she reminded herself that it wasn't any scarier than nine, and nine wasn't any scarier than ten. She was breaking the feeling of being out of control and gave herself permission to feel scared during the next mile. While she felt the fear, her knee went back to normal.

She finally figured out why she had this phantom knee problem. In the future, she would just acknowledge it and ask herself why she was afraid, and the feeling of pain and anxiety would relax.

She looked up from staring at the ground just in time to run past mile marker NINE and another hilarious sign that read, "Smile if you peed a little," which made her grin. The group near the sign was clapping for each and every one of the runners, and Lindsey thought to herself that everyone should run at least one race in their life. Where else could you get perfect strangers cheering you on and yelling your name? It was truly a memory she was etching into her brain for the future days when her life would be hard, and there would be no one around to yell, "You've got this!"

A few minutes after the excitement from the crowd, Lindsey hunkered down in her own space and focused on her red running shoes. She immediately saw a long yellow line on the ground, the center lane of the closed-off street. Her field of vision was just the yellow line, and in her mind, she imagined she was a tightrope walker. Could she keep her feet on the line without falling to her death? This became the game she started to create in her mind. Stay on the line, and she would make it across. She could see the line getting bigger and bigger, and her imagination took her from high-rise buildings to Niagara Falls. She was the famous tightrope walker who had mastered it all. She heard the clapping and encouragement in the distance and snapped out of her make-believe life.

She had managed to run past mile markers TEN and ELEVEN while she was tightrope running. She was glad the race had signs and volunteers directing the runners, because if she had been in the woods, she would have been completely lost after those two miles.

The sun was shining directly on her face as she squinted ahead. She unclipped her visor from her running belt and fastened it on her head. Lindsey had to pull out her ponytail since it was all jacked up and readjust it with the visor at an angle. She became aware that her arms were tired from running and redoing her hair. For the next few minutes, she shook her arms to her sides to get some stiffness out of them. She must have been running with her arms too tense at her elbows because she started to notice her shoulders were tight as well. Now, she was conscious of her whole back being stiff. She imagined how good it would feel to get a massage at the end of the race. Too bad she wasn't running the half marathon, she thought. She'd be close to that celebratory massage in a few miles.

This led her to darker thoughts about quitting again. Lindsey just wanted to stop running. She wanted that massage now. She wanted a glass of champagne. She wanted hugs from her family and friends. She wanted a kiss from John.

She wanted... She wanted to stop thinking this way. She pulled her granola bar out of her zipped pouch and started munching on it while she ran. This was helping her get out of her mood. She could do this. She had already run twenty miles before. This is fun. Well, she was trying to convince herself that this was fun, and up ahead, she made it to mile marker TWELVE.

CHAPTER FORTY-EIGHT

At mile marker twelve, Lindsey was feeling the festive activity all around her. The band at this mile seemed louder and much more fun. There were way more spectators and volunteers all clapping and encouraging the runners.

A few of the volunteers were in the center of the street, standing on Lindsey's tightrope. Those volunteers were directing the half marathoners to veer off to the left up ahead as they were close to finishing their race. Lindsey thought for a moment how great it would be to be finished with the race but kept focusing on the running.

As she ran closer to the split-off for the marathoners, there were more volunteers yelling out directions for the half marathoners to go to the left. They were congratulating and clapping loudly for the half marathoners.

They were continuously yelling through microphones, "Half marathoners to the left, marathoners stay on the right." All Lindsey kept thinking they were saying as they repeated the same sentences over and over were, "Half marathoners to the left, crazy people to the right," "Half marathoners, you are finished, marathoners, you have a long way to go," "Half marathoners, you are awesome, marathoners, keep running, you idiots."

It was all of these weird combinations of words said in Lindsey's mind that had half marathoners being smart because they were finishing and marathoners being dumb because they signed up for more punishment. She saw so many of the runners that she had been running with for the past few hours veer off to the left. They were soon to be done, and she had another half marathon to go.

She was noticing fewer and fewer runners continuing on and ran past mile marker THIRTEEN. This is when the tears started to form in her eyes. She was crying—crying for all of the months of training and hard work, crying because she was afraid, crying for signing up for the full marathon.

The crying turned into sobbing. At this point, she didn't even care if anyone was around or how she was acting. She was sobbing about everything. She was thirty-one. She hadn't really traveled anywhere. She didn't own a home. She wasn't married. She was tired. She was afraid of street lights swaying. She didn't take out the trash at her apartment last week, and it was probably smelling. She wanted to get a dog. She hated her car. She was too conservative. She wanted to dye her hair. She wanted to love with total abandon. She was angry at some of her customers.

She was getting hysterical and kept up the tears as she passed mile marker FOURTEEN. She was still weeping, but it automatically switched to the good things in her life. She was sobbing for getting to mile fourteen. She was crying for her best friend Ida. She was happy crying that she really loved John and was going to tell him. She felt empowered at her job. She was strong. She was amazing. She was resilient. She could and would do this marathon.

Lindsey ran out of tears. The crying really did wonders. Her sobbing moved to short, measured breaths to finally deep breaths of release. She was coming up on mile marker FIFTEEN as she wiped her face just in time to see her family hooting and hollering her name. She was going to be fine. She was already feeling much better, and her family was the icing on the cake.

The group was getting pretty rowdy and hugging Lindsey extra hard. She saw that John and her dad were the only sober ones in the group. It was like they were rounding up a herd of cattle, and she wished them luck. Ida tried to get Lindsey to drink from the new bottle of champagne as she passed, but Lindsey thought better of it since she still had eleven-plus miles to go. John gave a big hug, and that hug felt like an energy surge that would propel Lindsey to get to the next meetup point at mile twenty-two.

Aunt Joann jumped out into the street with Lindsey and started to walk with her while she drank her water for about a quarter mile with her. She was going on and on about how Lindsey has inspired the whole family to push themselves and venture out of their comfort zone. She even mentioned that she and her sisters were all going to take an *Authentically You!*® course from the lady that they had experienced reiki with the day before.

Lindsey was shocked and amazed that her running could get her aunts to discover themselves and actually take a self-help course. Her mother was actually taking an *Authentically You!* course? Was this the twilight zone?

As Lindsey ran off on her own towards mile sixteen, she went over in her head those words said by her aunt. She was surprised that her running had again made a difference in someone else's life. Her mom and sisters were going to take a course on being authentic? They were all going to find themselves now in their fifties and sixties? She started to laugh because she realized it didn't matter when you found yourself. It mattered that you wanted to find yourself, and getting to know the real you was the greatest find ever.

As she continued on and passed mile marker SIXTEEN, she knew she was learning about her whole being on this race and transforming into her own authentic self.

CHAPTER FORTY-NINE

As Lindsey continued toward mile seventeen, she noticed a guy in a bright green and red shirt walking ahead of her. It looked like a soccer jersey, though she couldn't say for sure since she didn't know much about soccer. The shirt had the word "CALIENTE" printed in large letters. She remembered from high school Spanish that it meant "hot" or "spicy." Her classmates used to use it jokingly to describe attractive guys. Smiling at the thought, Lindsey was reminded of her own "caliente" man back at mile fifteen. He was definitely hot!

She turned up her music just in time to hear *Joy and Pain*. The song made her giggle, taking her back to her college days. She and her roommates used to drink tequila and play that song before heading out for a night on the town. It was all joy while drinking the tequila, and pain the next day.

This race, too, was a mix of joy and pain, sunshine, and thankfully, no rain. The song lifted her spirits, so she put it on repeat as she pushed past mile marker SEVENTEEN.

By now, Lindsey had perfected her strategy for the hydration stations—knowing when to grab a drink and when to skip. Mile seventeen was a water stop, so she grabbed a bottle and swallowed another salt packet. This time, she didn't even bother opening it. Her confidence in managing the race was growing, though so was her bladder.

The need to pee was becoming an unavoidable thought. She vaguely remembered passing some porta-potties a few miles back but couldn't recall exactly where. She knew she'd have to find the next one soon and stop, no matter what. The race was inching closer to the finish line, and she couldn't risk there being no more stops ahead.

Keeping her eyes peeled for a porta-potty, Lindsey noticed the *caliente* guy running past her on her left. Wait—wasn't he walking earlier? She couldn't let someone who'd been walking overtake her, so she picked up her pace. The sudden movement jostled her stomach, making the situation more urgent. Finding a bathroom was now her top priority, even if it meant letting the *caliente* guy get ahead of her.

Finally, she spotted a porta-potty up ahead but groaned when she saw the line—at least six people were waiting. Lindsey joined the queue, shifting her weight and moving her legs to keep them loose while desperately trying to hold in the pressure.

As she waited, she noticed some runners slipping around to the back of a nearby industrial building and returning only moments later. Among them was the *caliente* guy. That was all the motivation she needed. Lindsey stepped out of line and followed the others to the back of the building, where she found two other women squatting. They were laughing and motioned for her to join them.

Desperate, Lindsey did just that, but what she hadn't antici-pated was how difficult it would be to stand back up. Her "marathon legs" were locking up in the crouched position, and now she understood why the other women were laughing.

From the sounds of their loud laughter and inappropriate jokes, Lindsey could only imagine what the people waiting in line for the porta-potty must have thought. Finally, after a lot of effort and some awkward shaking to minimize the damage to her running gear, Lindsey managed to shimmy up the wall and stand. She wished the other women good luck and ran off, determined to catch up to the *caliente* guy.

CHAPTER FIFTY

Lindsey was blown away up at mile EIGHTEEN. Her emotions got the best of her as she found a few more tears that she thought she had used up way back at mile thirteen through fifteen. There was a group and tent specifically for the first-time green bib marathoners. They had all kinds of signs and were individually saying Lindsey's name and making a point to call out how special she was as a first-timer.

It was perfect timing to have those particular volunteers at that spot. Lindsey was extremely glad for that encouragement. Her legs were starting to feel like jello, and the chafing under her left boob was irritating. She was running in the hard section where it was mostly industrial buildings and cement, with nothing to really look at besides the spectators.

As Lindsey continued on, she wondered what was really the reason she started running. At first, she wanted to find a way to work out without running into her ex, but that had quickly changed the first few times she started to run. She perceived that it became more about pushing herself to uncomfortable situations to help her grow. She noticed that the time alone helped her become a cheerleader of sorts to herself. She was finding out that she was stronger than she ever imagined. She could quiet her mind and allow her intuition to propel her forward.

She was also helping motivate others in finding themselves as well. She thought about her mother and how, in this process of running, she put herself first and set boundaries. She wasn't going to dwell on the past but look to the present, at how her mother was inspired to also grow. Maybe she finally would have a relationship that would be equal in love and encouragement. Running took a lot out of her, but it also gave so much in return.

She was taking this time to appreciate all that she had learned, and in that process, she noticed she had caught up to *caliente* guy and was passing him at mile NINETEEN. He was again walking, and she wondered what was going on in his head. She sipped on some electrolyte from her running belt and continued on.

The joy of passing him slowly vanished as she was starting to feel tired. She had music on, but it wasn't motivating her. She saw up ahead a man with a shirt that read, "I don't do marathons, I do a marathon runner." Lindsey chuckled to herself and thought that would be a great T-shirt for John. Lindsey wasn't sure if he would wear it, but she promised to at least tell him about the shirt if her runner's brain could remember.

She skipped ahead a few more songs until she got a Black Eyed Peas song that helped energize her. Turning up the volume, she started to clap her hands to will herself forward. It was going to be a bunch of mind games to get to the finish, and clapping her hands was working. It was also making her hands feel needed. She had been running so long with her fists clenched that the clapping was relaxing and relieving her tension.

She thought she probably looked ridiculous, but she was

running a marathon, and anyone at that stage in the race probably looked out of sorts. So she continued clapping all the way to mile TWENTY.

Around mile twenty, her mind went to everything that she was going to eat later. She was thinking about salty chips. Did John have any salty chips at home? Would she need to have him stop at the store? Was salt and vinegar chips what she really wanted, or maybe it was chips with dip? Tortilla chips with guac and salsa sounded good as well. Not those lime-flavored ones, but the traditional chips that were the restaurant style—the perfect ones for dipping.

She thought about other salty things, such as olives, as well. She loved garlic olives and blue cheese olives too. Blue cheese olives were perfect for her dirty martini. God, she would love a dirty martini. Only one, though, because those were always her downfall, and a second one just led to no good. But could she stop at one martini today? Probably not. So, dirty martinis were out of the question.

She was thinking of other salty drinks just as the *caliente* guy again was passing her. This guy was pissing her off. How could he be walking and then just pass her again? She turned her energy toward trying to keep up with him as he ran faster and faster. He was running too fast, and she couldn't keep up. The anger was rising in her as he continued to run further and further into the distance.

CHAPTER FIFTY-ONE

She came up to mile marker TWENTY-ONE and still no sight of the hot and spicy guy. *How much further ahead was he?* she thought to herself. She was passing quite a few other runners in the marathon and noticing their faces of defeat. They were fighting their own battles, and she was trying to stay ahead of her own. Her only solace was that her family was at mile marker twenty-two, so she only had to get to that mile for more encouragement.

This race was an eye-opening experience. She was at the point where she had never in her life run this far. She felt like she was cliff diving with no end in sight. Her own motivation could only carry her so far—she needed others too. This was a lesson on life as well.

Lindsey started to make up stories about the runners and spectators to quell her mind. She decided that the person running in front of her was stuck in a dead-end job at the Secretary of State's office, fielding complaints on wait times and handling license plate renewals. The disheveled body stance made it even more believable in Lindsey's mind. She envisioned this woman had to run in order to stay sane and that she was one mile away from cracking under pressure at work. She fantasized about how many kids she had at home and even what she had named them. George was named after her grandfather on her father's side, and they called him Georgie. He was probably on the race course with a sign that read, *"Go Mom."*

She thought about her own ideas on kids. Would she want one or two? Funny thing about that—she wanted kids with her ex, and it was probably to make him happy. Since she was always trying to please him, kids would have been a temporary fix for a while, but it wouldn't have made their relationship better. When she really thought about it, she wondered if she wanted them at all.

Her thoughts about children dwindled as she began searching for her family and friends. She was at mile TWENTY-TWO, and she couldn't see her family. *Where were they?* She was starting to stress out that her family wasn't where they said they would be. It was mile twenty-two, and there was no sight of them at all. To make matters worse, the *caliente* guy was still ahead of her.

She stopped at the water station and walked through, taking some sips of the water handed to her. She tried not to get discouraged. *Maybe my family is at another mile marker. Maybe I just got the numbers mixed up.* Quickly, she gulped the last sip and forged on to see if they were at the next mile.

The gulping of water was not a good idea, as Lindsey started to cough uncontrollably. She began hacking and hacking, just in time to look up and see her whole crew waving on the right side.

"Come on, girl, just swallow it! Everyone knows you just swallow it and don't spit. Are you choking on your own words?" It was Ida's voice yelling out inappropriate sayings to Lindsey. It was just like Ida to put Lindsey into a laughing, coughing spell, and her whole family was there to witness it.

John jumped out into the street to let Lindsey know that

parking was terrible and they had to park a bit past mile twenty-two. She was so happy at that very moment that she gave him a big kiss in front of everyone. Aunt Theresa was jumping up and down, yelling encouraging words. Lindsey knew it was the champagne talking and was amazed at her resilience after just losing her spouse.

She needed this family energy to lift her spirits, and they came through. She wanted to stop and just enjoy her family and friends, but she only had a few more miles to go, and she *had* to pass that caliente runner.

Off she went, with hooting and hollering in the background. It felt a little embarrassing to have all this attention, but it also felt really good. She turned right onto the street going into the last section of the race. It was the Victorian district with narrow streets and large, old mansions.

On each side of the street, there were house parties of all sorts. Lindsey had heard about this area being swanky and eclectic, and it definitely did not disappoint. The first house on the left had an entire jazz band, and everyone was dressed to the nines. It was practically a garden party with runners as the main event.

Over on the right was a group dressed as *Star Wars* characters. Lindsey assumed it was their version of alien chic and enjoyed trying to figure out who was the best dressed. They were giving out oranges to the runners, and Lindsey grabbed one for good measure.

Up ahead, she immediately recognized someone walking and picked up her stride. The *caliente* guy was eating an orange and walking. This was her moment to pass him again. She focused on her pace and form and immediately passed him on his right. It was about one hundred feet from mile TWENTY-THREE.

She turned up her music and enjoyed the surroundings,

knowing her family would be at the finish line and that she was ahead of the *caliente* guy.

CHAPTER FIFTY-TWO

A few minutes into the next song and just past mile TWENTY-THREE, Lindsey realized she only had a 5K left to run. *Only 3.1 miles left to finish this sucker.* It was an exciting thought—and a daunting one. How could she be so close to the end of a race and yet feel like it would never end?

Her mind drifted back to car rides with her parents when she was younger, driving up north to Aunt Theresa and Uncle Ned's place. It was always that last hour of the trip that felt the worst. She'd sit in the backseat, itching with anticipation for the lake and the water toys, only to feel trapped by her dad's slow driving, dragging out the journey even more.

Now, she was running that same metaphorical stretch of highway. She wanted so badly to get to the finish line, but her body felt like it was moving at her dad's speed. No matter how much she willed herself to push harder, she couldn't go any faster. It was like being stuck in that car all over again.

Her legs were stiffening with every step. She felt like the Tin Man from *The Wizard of Oz*. It was the oddest sensation—to want to run but feel her body resisting, like it wasn't entirely her own anymore. She reminded herself to lean forward in her stance, letting gravity do some of the work to propel her forward.

Ahead, she spotted a group of guys with a keg at the edge of the street in the Victorian district. They were handing out small cups of beer to runners. *Is that a good idea?* she wondered briefly. But as she slowed near them, the idea seemed more tempting. She grabbed a cup.

The beer was cold, refreshing, and delicious. A few sips were all she needed to feel a tiny spark of energy reignite within her. Somehow, she found herself running a little faster.

Lindsey couldn't help but wish there was more beer scattered along the last few miles of the course. She let her mind settle on the thought of running for beer. Yes, she would run for beer. She pictured an ice-cold pint waiting for her at the finish line, served in a frosty glass and paired with a tray of chips. *Yes, chips too,* she thought with a smile. The tray would be held by John, of course. That was an image she could get behind.

Her smile was quickly wiped away when, out of the corner of her eye, she saw the *caliente* guy passing her again.

Crap, she thought. *How is he doing this?* How could he walk earlier and still pass her now? Was she running that slowly? Irritation bubbled up inside her, momentarily overtaking her fatigue. She was so distracted by his sudden burst of speed that she almost didn't notice she had passed mile marker TWENTY-FOUR.

It was time to rally. Her Tin Man legs would have to work, whether they wanted to or not. There was no way she was going to let the *caliente* guy beat her.

No more stopping, she thought. Hydration stations were a thing of the past. The water in her belt would have to do. She clenched her jaw, shifted into determination mode, and set her sights on her newfound nemesis.

CHAPTER FIFTY-THREE

The fierceness in Lindsey's eyes kept her laser-focused. She was determined to pass the *caliente* guy at all costs. It felt strange how this random runner had become such a driving force for her. She was both grateful for him and annoyed by him. How odd it was, she thought, that competition could be both motivating and maddening.

Is he getting the best of me? she wondered. Lindsey reminded herself that this race wasn't about him. It was about *her*—her growth, her strength, and her determination. She was doing something no one in her family had ever done. She was learning to face her fears and push through them. This was more than just running; this was transformation.

In her mind, she pictured giving herself a hug. *You are strong. You are amazing.* This wasn't happening *to* her; it was happening *for* her. The *caliente* guy wasn't her enemy—he was her motivation. He was giving her a reason to dig deep and finish strong.

Up ahead, she saw him again. He was walking. *This is my chance,* she thought, straightening her form and quickening her pace. Mile TWENTY-FIVE loomed just ahead. Lindsey couldn't believe she had been running for five hours straight. That was like watching two movies back-to-back in a theater—but instead of sitting, she had been pounding pavement the entire time. She shook her head at the absurdity of it all. *No wonder I'm crazy enough to care this much about beating some random guy.* She ran by him this time on his left, thinking that would change her luck. She only had a little over a mile left, and it was so draining trying to stay ahead of him.

The last mile did sort of a loop near the finish line, and she happened to spot Ida all by herself running at Lindsey on the street. Ida was huffing and puffing and quite drunk. She insisted that she could run the last mile with her and help her finish. What Ida didn't know was that Lindsey was only worried about the caliente guy passing her. She would have to stay at a pace that would keep her in front.

Ida was so funny, and it was all Lindsey could do to not laugh. Ida ran in an odd way, barely keeping up. Here Lindsey was running her last mile, and Ida couldn't even run a quarter of it. It made her remember how her first days of running were so hard.

Lindsey turned down her music to let her friend know that she was proud of her running and that she could do it. Ida kept slowing down even with the encouraging words. This put Lindsey in a panic because the *caliente* guy was right next to her and Ida and was now passing her.

Lindsey told Ida she loved her and said she would see her at the finish. All she heard in the background was Ida heaving and yelling her name. She had to make sure this runner guy would not beat her as she left her best friend behind.

Lindsey turned up her music again. It was Elton John singing, "I'm still standing, yeah yeah yeah." How perfectly timed this song was, and she cherished all the selected songs that Ida had painstakingly planned for the race. This song was so true. She was still standing.

Mile marker TWENTY-SIX was coming upon them, and the

gated area was just in the distance. She could hear the announcer telling the time and names of some of the marathoners. She wondered if her name would be called since she was a first-timer.

She struggled to keep up with the caliente guy. He moved into a faster gear that made her feel like her legs were going to fall off. Could she even keep up with him? It was only POINT TWO left of the race, and her legs were turning into solid glue. She tried to hop-run and swung her arms harder and harder to keep up. She wanted to give up. The finish line was right in front of her, and she wanted to quit.

All of a sudden, she heard her name so loud as if it was the only name in the whole world. "Lindsey! Lindsey! Lindsey!" She saw the clock time and the finish line straight in front. She willed the last bit of energy she had and crossed the FINISH line.

She had no idea if she beat the *caliente* guy or if he finished before—it didn't matter anymore. She did it. She really did it. Her legs were literally about to fall off as the volunteers placed the alien-looking marathon medal around Lindsey's neck. She heard her name and a finish time that was muffled in her head and wobbled through the line, getting a race blanket draped over her as well.

There were all sorts of energy replenishments in the finish area and the holy grail of a massage tent. Lindsey grabbed half of a banana and dragged her legs over to the massage sign-up. The marathoners didn't have to wait, as there were plenty of amazing volunteers set up to give rubdowns on the runners' legs.

Lindsey fell forward on one of the tables and had the most relaxing and comforting 15-minute massage of her life. Running for this was definitely worth it, she thought. If it wasn't for the person tapping her that they were finished, she would have been passed out on the table for hours.

It was next to impossible to get up and move. Her knees were all locked up as she walked out to the greeting area. Her arms were coated in salt, and her crotch and breast area were completely rashy. She thought maybe she had a few blisters on her feet as well.

As she looked down at her phone, she noticed it was blowing up with texts of congratulations and support. There were texts from Brad, Mark, and Meg with fun emojis of runners and celebratory memes. They were all following along on the marathon app and could see that Lindsey had finished.

She hobbled out to find her supporters toward where they had texted and saw John with flowers. She saw her mom crying and Ida as well. It was funny to Lindsey because she had no more tears left. She left them all back at the race.

Her mom immediately hugged her and told her how proud she was. She was then tackled by Ida, who was still crying and also suggesting that they go get food ASAP. She had hugs from Aunt Joanne, who said she was so inspired by her running. She had kisses from Aunt Mary and Theresa, who congratulated Lindsey on an amazing accomplishment. Additional hugs were had by Lindsey's cousins and a big bear hug by her dad.

As Lindsey relished in all this love, she couldn't help but want to move to John, who was still holding flowers. John placed the flowers in Lindsey's arms and took them both into his. He had a few tears in his eyes as well as he whispered into her ear that he loved her too.

The words shocked Lindsey into reality as she realized John did hear her that one night when she said she loved him. She pulled back and sat down on the curb, overwhelmed at all the love and understanding of what had just occurred.

Ida sprang into action, pulling out the clean alien marathon shirt and flip-flops and the first-timer letters from everyone, and handed them to Lindsey. Lindsey slowly removed her sweaty running shirt with green bib numbers, leaving her with just her running bra, and put on her commemorative marathon shirt, making sure her medal still was facing the correct way. She pulled off her red running shoes and wet socks, finding all sorts of surprises on her feet, including at least two blisters, and slipped on the comforting slip-on shoes. She took the letters that were sitting in her lap from her friends and family and shoved them into her swag bag to read later.

Sitting on the curb, Lindsey took in the excitement of the after-party. She was surrounded by people who loved her. The same people who drank all of the celebratory champagne before she even finished. The same people who wanted to make changes to their lives as well. She was thankful for each of them.

The question was brought up again about where she wanted to go to eat, as everyone was starving. Lindsey knew she wanted something salty, like chips and a cocktail. She thought back to the one runner that helped push her—the *caliente* guy—and immediately the perfect idea appeared. "How about Mexican?" Lindsey asked. "And can someone help me up?"

ACKNOWLEDGMENTS

I would first like to thank my best friend, Cari Kussy, who inspired me to actually take my first steps of running outdoors - my husband, Sean Krabach, who supported me through it all - my father-in-law Larry Krabach who managed on many occasions to boat me over for my long runs, - my girlfriends – Nancy Uhl Curtis and Kristin Shust for actually wanting to take on running, immediately after my first marathon - Amanda Dana for finally inspiring me to finish this book and her wife, Jane Dana, for holding the both of us accountable to send her chapters.

I would also like to thank the motley marathon crew who came out for my first marathon in Detroit in 2008 – Wendy Krabach, Marsha Goode, Jennifer Bux, Michael Goode, Monique Goode, Sean Krabach, Cari Kussy, Jackie Goode, Gabe Goode, Larry Krabach

A FEW LETTERS FROM MY ACTUAL 1ST MARATHON

I have never been more proud of anyone than right now. I am so happy you have finished such an amazing goal! Blah – Blah – Blah – Blah ...

Seriously! Could you please run that faster next time? I mean it's cold here, my Arizona blood can't take it!

I honestly never thought a year ago – when I said – "The pavements free – go for a run" that we would be watching you run a marathon! It is so amazing! Everybody I tell can't believe it's <u>You</u> doing it! You have at least motivated me to do a 5k! (I gotta start small) Maybe there is a naked marathon you could do somewhere – or at least one in a thong! God, that image still kills me! Frankly, I wouldn't wear any underwear – I mean, what's the point anyway? God, the other day I had these thongs on and I swear I could feel them in my throat – That was a long day. Speaking of long days... how about today! I bet that feels like you ran a marathon! LOL! What are you going to do next? Grab some Pad Thai? And a beer? I don't actually drink beer – but I will be drunk probably by the time you are reading this anyway!

Enough about you – Let's talk about me! Do you think I should cut another inch off my hair? Does my skin look better? What should I wear tomorrow?

I honestly can't stop laughing. It's so hard to stop shaking and doing that internal laugh thing!

What the hell! I mean it's a fucking miracle! Really! Did you ever think in your wildest dreams you would run the Detroit marathon? I didn't. Until like 5 months ago when you went to Royal Oak to watch a movie about running – I was like – WOW. She is crazy! Nothing sounded boringer than running 26.2 miles til I hear there was a movie about running 26.2 miles.

At this point I have actually begun laughing right out loud – people are looking at me! This is great!

I love you so much. In total truth, you are my sister, my best friend, and more! You are my witness. Which is why there is <u>no way</u> I wasn't going to <u>witness This!</u>

I love you – I am so proud of you!

I admire you! So much!

All my love!

Cari

AKA – The Queen

October 19, 2008

Amy,

Well, you did "it"! By "it", I mean finished the marathon, or maybe I mean "tried the marathon", either way, it doesn't matter. You set a goal and worked for it.

I am so proud of you. I know you work really hard on your business, around the house and in everything you do. I also know I am sometimes hard on you and that it's unfair. I am trying to work on that.

Back to this running thing.

Not quite sure how you changed your mind, but I swear that when I ran the Turkey Trot way back when, you said no one in their right mind would ever do that and now, you are

the one that is crazy! I mean, who really wants to run 26.2 miles?

Did I tell you how proud of you I am? Oh yeah, I did that up above.

You convinced me to try it, so if you are looking for a running partner for next year, I'm in. I will run with you. You are going to have to help me with my training though. I don't think I can do it on my own.

Now that you are a runner, you are getting a hot runners body too! That's the best part for me. In the long run, it probably just means that you will outlive me.

Once again, I am so proud of you.

Now that I am sure this running bug will go away, what do you want to do next? Maybe I'll try it too. Just nothing that involves spinning carnival rides.

So, if you finished the whole 26.2 miles, congratulations! I can't believe it. If you didn't do the whole thing, so what. You tried and I love that you have the desire and dare to try while many others don't. Keep up the hard work. I will always support you and most of all, I will always love you!

P.S. – That support thing is a spiritually not a financial thing.

SEAN.

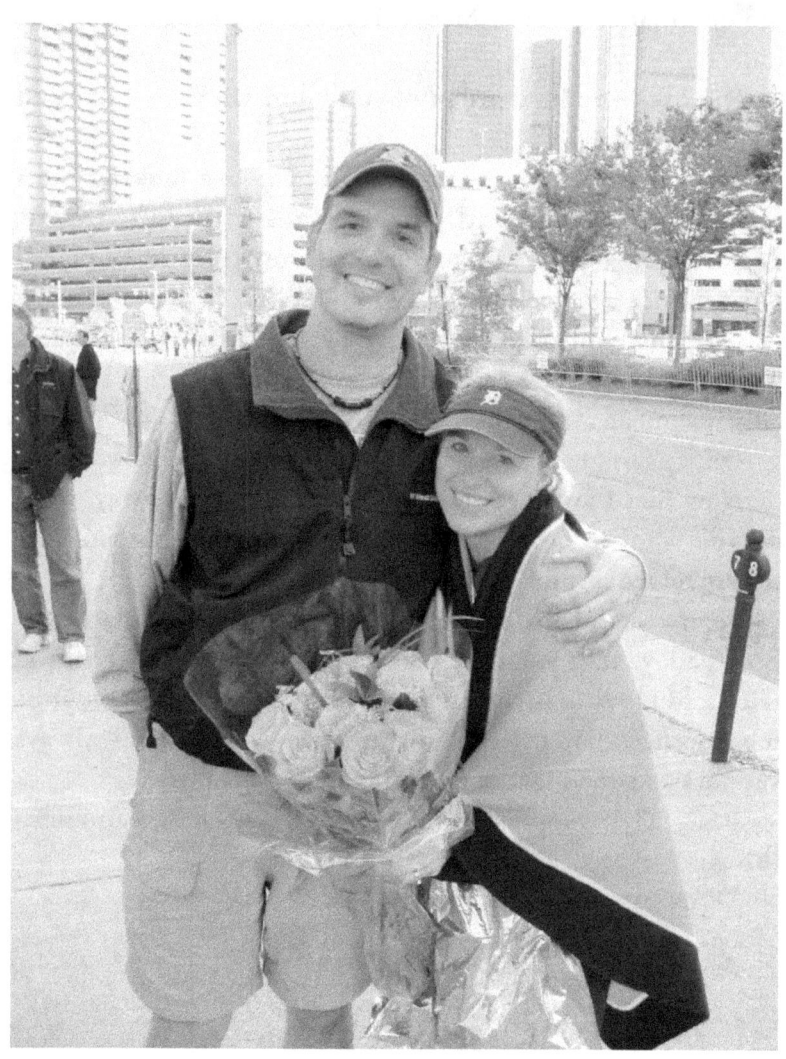

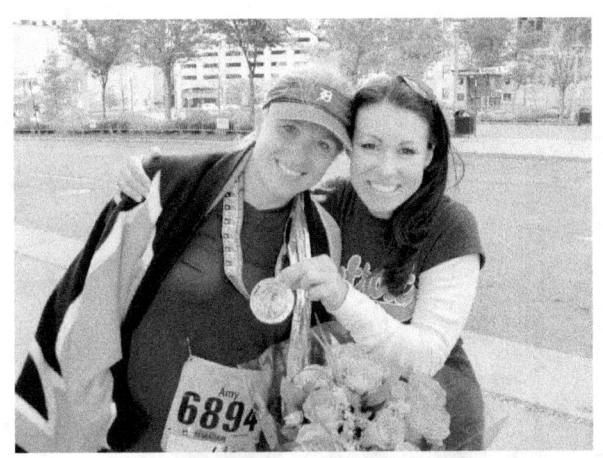

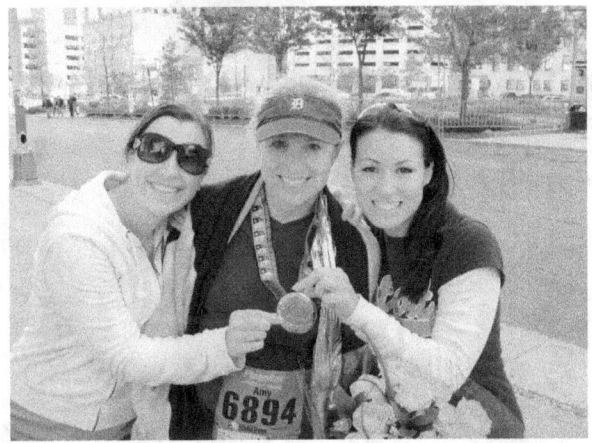

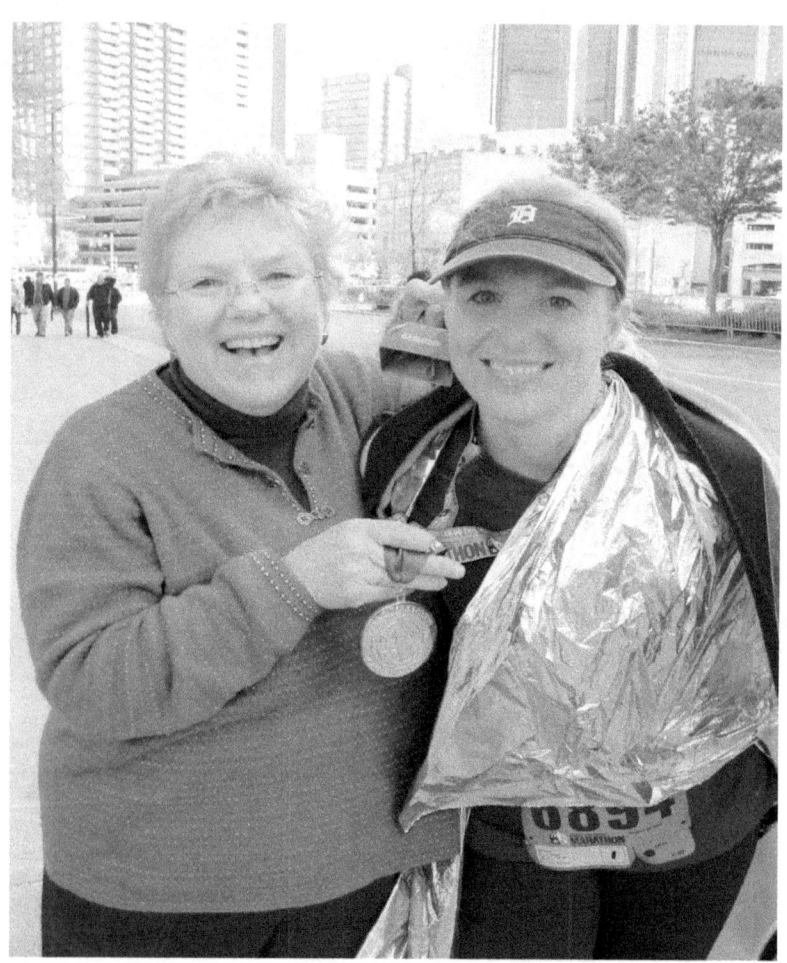

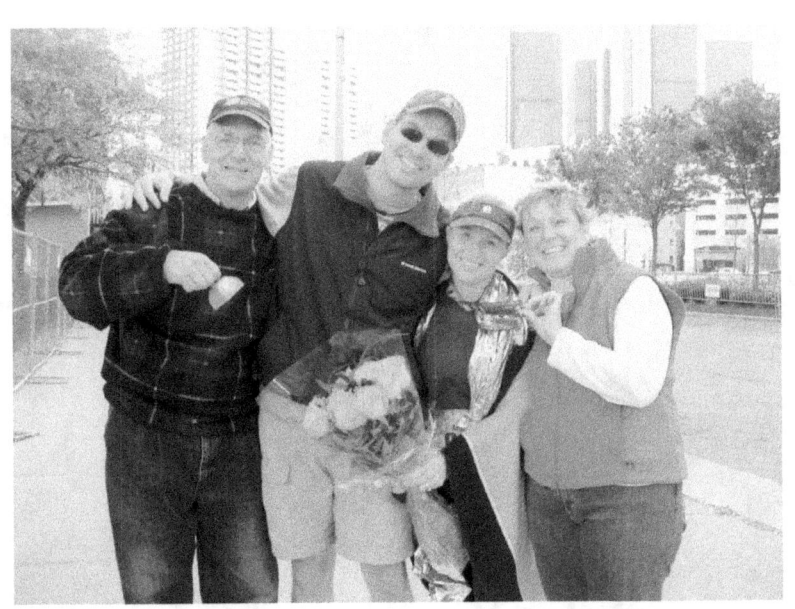

ABOUT THE AUTHOR

Amelia Krabach is a passionate healer, teacher, and guide on the journey to self-discovery. As the founder of Team You LLC and the visionary behind the *Authentically You!®* program, she has spent over two decades helping others align mind, body, and soul. A certified Reiki Master and Energy Worker, Amelia weaves together spiritual wisdom, emotional healing, and personal empowerment to support clients in becoming their truest selves.

Drawing from her own transformative experiences, *Running to You* is a heartfelt invitation to reconnect with the self you may have left behind or never knew at all. Amelia lives in Novi, Michigan, with her husband, Sean, their dog Finnegan, and their cat Benny. When she's not teaching or writing, you'll find her guiding others through deep inner work, supporting new healers, or exploring the mystical side of life. You may find more work and programs by Amelia at www.theteamyou.com

www.ingramcontent.com/pod-product-compliance
Lightning Source LLC
Chambersburg PA
CBHW071522100726
47908CB00004B/1257